CONQUERING YOUR CHILD'S ALLERGIES

M. Eric Gershwin, M.D.
Edwin L. Klingelhofer, Ph.D.

ADDISON-WESLEY PUBLISHING COMPANY, INC.

Reading, Massachusetts Menlo Park, California New York
Don Mills, Ontario Wokingham, England Amsterdam Bonn
Sydney Singapore Tokyo Madrid San Juan

Many of the designations used by manufacturers and sellers to distinguish their products are claimed as trademarks. Where those designations appear in this book and Addison-Wesley was aware of a trademark claim, the designations have been printed in initial capital letters (e.g., Tylenol).

Library of Congress Cataloging-in-Publication Data

Gershwin, M. Eric, 1946–
Conquering your child's allergies / M. Eric Gershwin, Edwin L. Klingelhofer.
p. cm.
Includes index.
ISBN 0-201-12967-1
ISBN 0-201-52340-X (pbk.)
1. Allergy in children—Popular works. I. Klingelhofer, E. L. (Ed. L.) II. Title.
RJ386.G47 1989
618.92'97—dc19 88-29248
CIP

Cover design by Hannus Design Associates
Cover photo by Bill Losh/FPG
Text design by Anna Post
Illustrations copyright © by Ruth Linstromberg
Set in 10-point Palatino by DEKR Corporation, Woburn, MA

ABCDEFGHIJ-DO-9543210
First printing, March 1989
First paperback printing, January 1990

This book is for our wives, Laurel and Jean, mothers who have dealt each day with their own children's allergies with incomparable understanding and patience.

To Our Readers

This book can help you and your family greatly. Its suggestions about health care reflect the best and most up-to-date medical information and opinion available. As with all medical advice, however, cases — and therefore treatments — may vary.

The authors and publisher therefore disclaim any responsibility for consequences resulting from following advice or procedures set forth in this book. It is not intended to be an alternative to or substitute for your own doctor's recommendations. In particular, the treatment of severe, protracted, or stubborn symptoms or the use of *any* drug or medication should be undertaken only after consultation with your own physician.

Acknowledgments

We are deeply indebted to the many people and organizations that helped us prepare this book. We particularly appreciate the help of

- The medical scientists who continue to further our understanding of allergies and render them more treatable in our patients.
- The American Academy of Allergy and Immunology and the American Lung Association and their chapters, as well as other groups and societies that responded to our numerous requests for information — particularly in compiling the information in the appendixes.

We owe special thanks to one person — Nikki Rojo, who typed this manuscript. Her enthusiasm, intelligence, and matchless skill really made the book happen. We also wish to thank Judy Van der Water for helping with the illustrations. Finally, we wish to thank Drs. Kenneth Epstein, Mark Fletcher, Maurice Hamilton, Donna Kinser, Stanley Naguwa, and Robert Teitscheid for reading and criticizing the text for us.

The mistakes that remain are ours alone.

M.E.G.
E.L.K.

Contents

Preface

The number of children with allergies is astounding — nearly one child in six is said to suffer from some sort of allergy. The problems of these allergic children can be as mild as occasional attacks of hay fever or as severe as disfiguring eczema and life-threatening bronchial asthma. In addition to the obvious health problems associated with having allergies, affected children may experience recurring colds, painful ear infections, and other allergy-linked conditions, all of which cause frequent school absences. Childhood allergies affect school performance adversely; they may be instrumental in reducing attention span, and they are certainly a major social, psychological, and financial burden for children and their parents.

This book is a complete guide to childhood allergies presented in simple, jargon-free language. It provides parents with comprehensive, up-to-date, and practical information and advice on how to help their allergic children. It identifies the many allergic symptoms, tells what they look like, how prevalent they are, what causes them, and what to do about them. It outlines steps parents can take to help their children understand, manage, and control their allergies. Its goal is to help parents and children cope effectively with a major childhood problem.

We wrote this book because we have had to live with allergies all of our lives, in ourselves and in our children. Both of us have had severely allergic children. We want to share with you what we have found out, and what Eric, who is a Professor of Medicine and Chief of Allergy, Rheumatology, and Clinical Immunology at the University of California, Davis, Medical School, teaches his medical students about caring for allergic children.

Introduction

Twentieth-century technology has dramatically improved virtually all aspects of medical treatment. Better prenatal care, improved hygiene and nutrition, the near-elimination of childhood diseases like polio and measles, the use of antibiotics to treat infections — these and many other developments have all contributed to better health and longer life.

Amidst these improvements we have also seen the emergence of allergies as one of the most common and troublesome health problems around. Childhood allergies are so widespread that nearly half of all families can point to at least one member whose life has been clouded by them. Allergies affect school achievement adversely and often bring on persistent, difficult to manage, and sometimes severe problems like poor appetite, sleep disturbances, irritability, and psychological disorders.

Bill, now in high school, had been troubled by recurrent colds, sore throats, and ear infections ever since he was a toddler. All through grade school he was academically below average and displayed little interest in his schoolwork. His parents felt that their doctor's office was their second home because of Bill's recurring and painful ear infections. Bill's father always wondered about the bluish discoloration under his son's eyes and mentioned it to a physician he saw while taking an insurance physical. The doctor suggested that Bill's eye discoloration might be a condition called "shiners" and that he might be suffering from allergies. The parents took Bill to an allergist who told them that Bill was severely allergic to house dust. The dust allergy had caused chronic irritation of the nasal membranes, stoppage of the eustachian tube, and infection-caused earaches. Bill's parents bought an air cleaner and took drastic precautions to make their home and car as dust-free as possible. The results were little short of amazing. One year later Bill's school performance had improved enough to put him in the top half of his class, and he became a serious, hard-working student.

Allergic children must be given special care. They have the same abilities and potential as other children, but their capacity to realize them to the fullest can be blocked by allergic diseases like severe hay fever, chronic eczema, or life-threatening asthma. The questions we must ask are

- How do we manage these special children?
- How can you, the parent, be sure your child's problems are *really* due to allergies?
- What are the telltale signs you should watch for in caring for your allergic child?
- Do allergic diseases have any special features that you need to be alert to?
- How are allergies treated? What can be done to manage allergies better or eliminate them?
- Do all doctors treat allergies in the same way? How do you find a doctor who will help you deal effectively with your child's allergies?
- What can you do to help your allergic child — and all of the other members of the family, *including yourself* — to lead a normal life?

We have written this book to answer these and other questions about childhood allergies. You will see that this book is unlike other books on allergy. Its language is simple and as free as possible of medical terms. It contains charts to help you decide, step by step, what you should do about specific signs and symptoms you see in your child. Above all, it strives to show you how you can take greater responsibility for the knowledgeable, effective, and aggressive management of your child's symptoms. This skillful management can minimize or totally eliminate the possible lifelong negative effects that neglected or poorly treated allergies can cause.

The book is divided into four sections. Part I is a brief introduction to what allergies are all about and what they mean to you and your child; Part II consists of six chapters which identify the causes or triggers of allergies or allergylike symptoms and the steps you can take to avoid or control them effectively. Part III contains 12 chapters devoted to the more common allergic symptoms and the measures you can take to detect, identify, manage, and relieve them. These symptoms represent the most common ones encountered in children; they are either allergy-caused or often blamed on allergies. Because some substances may provoke a variety of symptoms (pollens can be responsible for hay fever and asthma *and* make eczema worse, for instance), the connection between allergic symptoms and causes is complex and sometimes difficult to trace. Table 1 gives the bodily systems or areas most commonly affected by allergies, names the causes, lists the common symptoms they provoke, and cites the chapters in this volume that cover them. This table will help you to use the book efficiently.

The four chapters of Part IV dwell on how you can see to it that your child has the most effective long-term care. It deals with such important matters as how to choose a doctor and the role of vaccines, allergy tests, and immunization. It also covers the pitfalls to avoid in maintaining effective treatment for allergies, alerts you to some special problems and dangers that common illnesses represent to allergic youngsters, offers suggestions as to how the morale and psychological well-being of the allergic child — and you, the caring parent — can be kept high, offers a prescription for living as close to a normal life as possible with allergies, discusses the special duties and obligations associated with parenting allergic children, and tells parents what to expect over the long haul.

Nan well exemplifies what parents can do to help an allergic child.

> Each weekday morning, Nan, a hard-working junior high school teacher, leaves her three-year-old daughter Jenny at the day care center near her home. Jenny is always fine when she is dropped off, but when her mom returns to pick her up, Jenny invariably has a severe runny nose and itchy eyes. Nan has tried a whole variety of medications; none seems to be effective. Moreover, she is puzzled because Jenny recovers so quickly on weekends. Nan had allergies when she was a child but Jenny seems free of them. Finally, in desperation, Nan consulted an allergist who suggested that Jenny might have an allergy to something in the day care center. Nan sat in with Jenny at the center and saw that Jenny had become extremely friendly with the owner's long-haired Burmese cat. Nan could not believe Jenny had an allergy to cats because they themselves have a cat who lives out-of-doors. Nan quickly changed her mind when Jenny started sneezing immediately after stroking and petting the cat.

Yet there are many pitfalls for parents along the way. There are hundreds of products sold either over-the-counter in the pharmacy or through magazines that are claimed to help children's allergies. Some of these are medications; others may be expensive (but not necessarily effective) air cleaners, vacuum cleaners, and other allergy-protective devices. While these products are well-intended and possibly helpful, they can be costly mistakes for parents faced with an acutely ill child.

When choosing a doctor, parents bear the ultimate responsibility for selecting someone who can provide the best care for their youngster. Who should it be? What questions should you ask? These and other medical matters should be addressed carefully by every parent and are discussed in later chapters.

Finally, and importantly, there is the matter of prevention. It is far easier to prevent the symptoms of allergies than to treat them once they appear. Being able to recognize telltale signs, being able to diagnose correctly, and being able to work with your doctor are all important tactics that we will emphasize throughout the book.

You, as a parent, will have to make some complex and difficult decisions. But the bottom line is that if you make them promptly, knowledgeably, and with the right kind of help, your child will benefit immeasurably.

TABLE 1 Classification of Allergic Diseases

SYSTEM OR AREA OF BODY AFFECTED	CAUSES	SYMPTOMS: MORE COMMON	SYMPTOMS: LESS COMMON	CHAPTERS
Gastrointestinal tract	Food Food additives	Colic (infants) Diarrhea Constipation Stomachache	Hives Asthma/wheezing Shock (anaphylaxis)	4,10
Respiratory tract	Pollens	Hay fever (seasonal) Itchy eyes (seasonal) Asthma	Earache	6,11,12,15,16
	Dust Mold Animal dander	Hay fever (chronic) Itchy eyes (chronic)	Asthma Earache	6,11,12,15,16
	Pollutants (smog, tobacco smoke, etc.)	Asthma Itchy eyes		6,11,15
	Infections (colds, flu)	Asthma	Hives	5,11,14,20
	Insect stings or bites	Hives	Wheezing	9,11
	Vigorous exercise, cold, dry air	Asthma	Shock	7,11
Skin	Plants Chemicals	Allergic contact dermatitis		8,17
	Unknown	Eczema		13
	Food or food additives	Hives		14
	Insect stings or bites Infection	Hives		9
Vascular system (blood pressure, pulse, etc.)	Food or food additives	Faintness, dizziness	Shock	4
	Medications	Faintness, dizziness	Shock	4
	Insect stings or bites	Pain	Shock	9
Psychological	Chronic illness Hyperventilation	Anxiety stress, depression, wheezing, headache		11,21,22

PART ONE

WHAT ARE ALLERGIES, WHY DO CHILDREN HAVE THEM, HOW CAN I BE SURE MY CHILD IS REALLY ALLERGIC, AND HOW CAN I BEST COPE WITH THE SITUATION?

1.

Why My Child?

When a child is diagnosed as having an allergy, a parent is likely to ask the doctor "Why my child?" One of the main reasons for the question stems from the fact that allergies, despite being commonplace, are not very well understood; there is probably more misinformation circulating about allergies than there is solid fact. One of the more persistent bits of misinformation is the belief that allergies are psychologically caused, that they are "all in the head" as the saying goes, and that the parent is somehow to blame for the sick child. When a parent asks "Why Janie?" he or she really wants to know, "What did I do to cause this suffering, and what can I do to prevent it?"

Allergies, despite the misinformation that surrounds them, are not psychologically caused, are not brought on by bad parenting or something equally dire.

More than 35 million Americans, adults and children, have allergies. No population in the world is allergy-free, although there are striking differences in the incidence and severity of allergies among them. In West Africa and among Native Americans, asthma is quite rare; in the British West Indies, nearly one third of the inhabitants have it.

In this country, residents of rural areas are more likely to have allergies, probably because they run into more allergens than city dwellers. Some ethnic groups, notably American blacks, also show higher rates of allergic disease.

The tendency to develop allergies is inherited or hereditary. However, there are also environmental or acquired influences. The hereditary basis has been established in several ways. Depending on the specific allergic complaint, a child whose parents are allergic is two to five times more likely to develop an allergy than a child whose parents are free of symptoms. Other studies have shown that if one member of a pair of identical twins has an allergy, the other twin will almost certainly develop it. On the other hand, nonidentical twins, even though they share the same environment, are not nearly as likely to share the same allergy.

Whether or not your child develops an allergy depends, in the final analysis, on whether or not your child is exposed to its cause. If your child is genetically disposed to react allergically to penicillin, he or she will develop this reaction only if penicillin is administered; even if there is inherited sensitivity to ragweed, a French child would not develop hay fever to ragweed, simply because ragweed does not grow in France. However, if the family emigrated to Michigan, the child would show hay fever symptoms within a few years.

Allergies can have much more serious physical consequences in children than they do in adults. For example,

- Asthma is much more prevalent and severe — in some instances life-threatening — in children.
- Eczema, an extremely uncomfortable and hard-to-manage complaint, very often starts in early childhood.
- Nasal allergies trigger serious, recurring ear infections and chronic headaches in many youngsters.
- The medications — especially those used to treat asthma — can be disagreeable to take and the side effects can be anything from unpleasant to dangerous. Nonetheless, when used properly medications can be wonderfully beneficial.
- Allergies can exert profound effects on the life of the child.
- Allergies are often responsible for extended and frequent school absences and poor school performance.
- Chronic allergies can have diffuse and troublesome psychological consequences, impairing normal development and adjustment and causing difficulty and handicaps in later life.
- Unless you are prepared, children chronically ill with allergies can play havoc with your and other family members' lives. Their care, which can be quite demanding and expensive, can preempt other considerations and disrupt normal family activities and relationships.

These problems are also compounded by the characteristics of the children as they pass through developmental stages. *During infancy* parents sense that something is the matter, but because of the inability of the child to communicate or complain they have no idea of the nature of the trouble.

In early childhood the ability to communicate improves but may be accompanied by confusion, little or no comprehension of what is happening, and the formation of stubborn or ineradicable fears or aversions to treatment, especially when it comes to taking unpleasant-tasting medicines or having shots.

In later childhood and adolescence, self-knowledge grows, and with this, some sense of how to cope with the complaint, whatever it is. The bad news is that at this stage the need to be like other children intensifies, and with it there is a strong tendency to resist measures of avoidance or treatment intended to manage the allergy. Sometimes kids seem to prefer risking illness to being seen as different or conspicuous when avoiding pollens or publicly using an asthma inhaler during an attack.

Penny, 14, hates being an asthmatic and goes to painful lengths to conceal her condition from her peers. She believes being seen using her Alupent inhaler would give away her secret, so she goes to great trouble never to use it in public. What happens, though, is that when she begins wheezing in class it soon gets to the point where everyone in the room hears her wheezing and is troubled by her struggle for breath. Her asthma is the worst-kept secret in the high school.

Finding out as much as you can about the condition, its cause, treatment, consequences, and how it is linked to other childhood illnesses, allergic and otherwise, will help you and your child cope with the problem and steer clear of hazards down the road. Eczema, for instance, most often turns up in infants. It is a distressing but easily treatable complaint which, if addressed promptly and competently, will leave no psychological or physical scars. It is likely to be followed by other allergic problems in childhood — asthma and hay fever particularly — and the informed parent will know what steps to take if these conditions do turn up. By recognizing these possibilities, many of the tribulations associated with allergies — such as visits to a series of specialists, conflicting diagnoses and the confusion that attends that, expense, and school absence — can be avoided. Good parents, good drivers, good ball players have this in common — they know what they will do in the event something happens, and they are prepared to do it the moment the anticipated situation develops.

Jason has had eczema from the time he was six months old. His mother has scrupulously avoided using soaps and she keeps his skin as moist and as lubricated as possible. Jason is now 11 years old and for the past three or four weeks his eczema has obviously gotten worse. His mother is perplexed as to what is happening. She is convinced she is doing everything right but missing a clue. Deciding to play Sherlock Holmes, she tracks and follows Jason throughout the day. After four days, she can find nothing whatsoever to point to as the source of the trouble, so she speaks to his pediatrician. He asks her about her laundry detergent. Jason's mom says that she has been using only about one quarter the recommended amount of laundry detergent on Jason's clothes and has not changed her method of washing in many years. However, the question about detergent reminded her that she had recently started using a fabric softener. (She thought the fabric softener would soften Jason's clothes and make them less harsh to his skin.) She had completely forgotten this change in routine because she started the fabric softener some two months before Jason's skin began to worsen. Jason's doctor has not heard of an allergy to fabric softener but advises her to discontinue using it, which she does. Within two weeks Jason's skin returns to its earlier state — readily managed mild eczema.

Parents with allergic children have the additional burden of having to learn and adhere conscientiously to treatment procedures for their child's complaint. They should know how to avoid and control exposure to triggers that cause allergies to develop, and they should encourage and assist the child to pursue as close to a full, normal, autonomous life as possible. Parents should continually remind themselves that

- At some time or another, allergies are found in most families.
- Allergies and asthma are not psychologically or emotionally caused.
- It is not the child's fault that he or she is allergic. Inner force or strength of character or resolve will not make the allergy vanish.
- Correct medications, properly taken, will usually improve but not "cure" allergies.

On the up side,

- Allergies are not catching.
- Most allergies do improve as children grow older; happily their physiology changes and they become easier to treat.
- Allergic children, with proper guidance, can do most everything other children do, including physical education in school, summer camp, and serious, even (given the talent) world-class, athletics.
- Allergies can be kept from dragging down school academic performance or interfering with the joy and excitement of growing up.
- Effective management of allergies in children is possible with sensible, informed, perceptive, alert, conscientious parents.

WHAT IS AN ALLERGY?

An allergy is a unique response by your body to a foreign material. Most often this response is to things we inhale, like pollen, dust, and animal dander, or things we swallow, like food. Our environment contains millions of germs or infectious agents — bacteria, viruses, mold — that could produce serious infections if they were to enter the body.

Our immune system blocks this invasion. There are also infectious agents called parasites. We do not hear much about parasites anymore, since modern hygiene has dramatically reduced their incidence in Western society. There was a time when parasites, such as worms, were common, particularly in warm or temperate climates where people went barefoot and worms entered the body from the earth via the skin of the feet.

One method that our body uses to fight such parasites is to release a special antibody known as immunoglobulin E, or IgE. This antibody is ordinarily present in very small concentrations. However, after the body is invaded by worms the antibody level rises, killing and preventing the spread of the invaders.

With the drop in incidence of parasites in the U.S., IgE is not really needed anymore. Although pinworms are still encountered occasionally in children, tapeworms, roundworms, and others are rare. Nonetheless, our capacity to make IgE evolved, and it continues to exist in all of us. Allergies are an unfortunate by-product of this IgE system. What happens is that our body, when it encounters pollens, animal dander, or other irritating substances, treats them like worms by producing a lot of IgE. Once IgE is produced, it travels through the blood and lodges on certain white cells, which are known as mast cells or basophils. While resting on these cells, IgE is harmless. However, if a person is exposed to pollen, animal dander, or dust at a time when the IgE is resting on white cells, dramatic events happen. The contact of the pollen with the IgE on white cells triggers a reaction. The white cells release certain chemicals, one of which is histamine. Histamine can cause sneezing, flushing, itching, and wheezing. In heavy enough doses it can cause severe or even deadly reactions. An allergic or atopic reaction, then, occurs in the following way:

1. A foreign substance invades the body and causes it to produce IgE.
2. The immune system (IgE) detects the presence of the invader and releases histamine and other chemicals from the white cells.
3. When enough chemicals from inside the white cells are released, the allergic symptoms occur locally — on the skin or in the respiratory, vascular, or digestive systems.

Most people do not have allergies, mainly because they do not produce enough IgE. This fact puzzles parents who want to know *"Why my child?"*.

Bob Brown is 11 years old and his brother Joey is 9. They are as alike as two brothers can be. Although Bob is taller, they could pass for twins. However, their health is very different. Bob suffers from recurrent allergies. It seems sometimes that he is allergic to everything — trees, grasses, pollens, weeds, molds, house dust, and many foods. Joey, on the other hand, is allergic to nothing. They both eat the same things. They grew up in the same house. They attend the same school. They like the same sports and hobbies. Bob, however, probably got his allergies by inheriting a special combined set of genes from both his mother and his father that allowed him to make more IgE than he should. Joey, on the other hand, did not inherit these types of genes and has always been spared from having allergies. The differences between most allergic and nonallergic children rest in their genes.

The fact that allergies are inherited does not mean that if you or your spouse had allergies, your child will necessarily have them. *Nor* does it mean that if you do not have allergies, your children will be spared. *Nor* does it mean that if one child has allergies another child will also turn up with allergies.

What it does mean is that you are more *likely* to see allergies in your children if one parent has an allergy. If both you and your mate have allergies, it is even more likely that your children will have allergies.

Another aspect of the allergy picture has to do with the differences between children and adults. Vulnerability to allergies depends on the age and level of maturation of the individual; children are more susceptible to them. Children are not small adults; they are developing and growing organisms. Many of their tissues and organs are not fully mature. Most materials that cause allergies are either inhaled or eaten. Thus, while children may ingest the same food that adults do, it is important to remember that their absorptive and digestive processes are different. In children, this immaturity often allows food materials to be absorbed and passed unchanged into the body, whereas in adults the food materials are digested more completely. Some foods, especially cow's milk, pass undigested into the bodies of children more easily than into the body of adults. In the case of the lungs, the airways are not fully mature in children and may permit pollen or other inhaled materials to get into the lungs more easily.

Finally, allergies that produce abnormalities of the skin, ears, nose, sinuses, or lungs may have widespread repercussions. Children with recurrent hay fever are more susceptible to earaches, ear infections, and sinus disease; children with asthma are more susceptible to bronchitis and pneumonia; children with eczema are more susceptible to many infections and diseases, including cataracts. Any chronically ill child is more susceptible to fatigue, tension, depression, restlessness, and sleep disorders. In short, taking care of allergic children involves much more than simply giving pills; it means *taking charge* as parents.

This book tells you how to take charge.

2.

How to Know if Your Child Is Allergic

The final decision on whether your child really has an allergy is for your doctor to make. Even so, there are a number of allergic signs that parents ought to recognize and report to the physician. They include:

- Do you, the parent, have a history of allergies?
- What exactly are the symptoms?
- When, where, and under what circumstances do symptoms show up and how do they manifest themselves?
- Are the symptoms associated with other factors you can point to like time of day, weather conditions, season of the year, being outdoors, particular foods, wearing apparel, medications, changes in personal habits, out-of-the-ordinary events?
- Are the symptoms attributable to an allergy or an allergy imposter?

FAMILY HISTORY OF ALLERGIES

The chances that a child will develop an allergy are greater if either or both of the parents have a history of allergies — two to five times greater, in fact. Thus, if the mother and the father have no history of eczema, the odds are approximately only 4 in 100 that their child will show this disease; if just the mother or the father has had eczema, there is about an 8% chance or better that the child will also experience it. The odds are greater, of course, if both parents have had the disease. Nevertheless, the chances of an allergic parent having an allergic child are slim. In addition, the appearance of symptoms, whatever they are, in the individual child is unpredictable. If the firstborn is allergic, that does not guarantee that succeeding children will automatically be so troubled.

Although heredity is a factor in the transmission of allergic diseases, its effect is not invariant, and except in the most extraordinary circumstances, allergic couples should not be too concerned about having allergic children. They should be aware of the risk, however, and prepared to furnish their physician with information about their allergic histories, and those of both sets of grandparents if that information can be obtained.

WHAT ARE THE SYMPTOMS?

Allergic symptoms most often involve the skin, the upper and lower respiratory systems, and the gastrointestinal tract. Less frequently (and usually as a companion to involvement of these major systems) they may turn up in the eyes, ears, or circulatory system.

The most common allergic symptoms and the organs or systems they affect are listed in Table 2; each of the associated allergic diseases is discussed in detail in the chapters that make up Part III of this book. Any of these complaints should alert you to the possibility that an allergy is implicated; if other, different symptoms are present in the systems listed, something other than an allergy is probably responsible.

THE WHEN AND HOW OF ALLERGIC DISEASES IN CHILDREN

Whether symptoms originate with an allergy depends to a considerable extent on the age of the child and the way in which symptoms show up and progress. Both of these aspects are dealt with comprehensively in the chapters making up Part III. Table 3 notes the typical age of onset and charts the usual course or progress for the most common allergic diseases in children.

ASSOCIATED FACTORS

Allergies can be tied to a host of factors or conditions — from the time of the year or the weather or what your child had for lunch to the arrival of a new pet, moving to a new house or apartment, using makeup, or even taking a walk in the country.

The most common of these allergy associates are named in the Al-

TABLE 2
Common Symptoms of Allergic Disease

ORGAN OR SYSTEM	*TYPE OF SYMPTOMS**	*POSSIBLE ALLERGIC DISEASE***
Skin	Sores	Eczema, contact dermatitis
	Wheals	Hives
	Intense Itching	Eczema, dermatitis, hives
Upper respiratory tract	Runny nose (clear, thin discharge)	Hay fever (seasonal or chronic)
	Sneezing, itchy throat	
Lower respiratory tract	Cough, thick clingy mucus, wheezing, shortness of breath	Asthma
Gastrointestinal tract	Stomachache Constipation Diarrhea Colic	Food allergy
Ears	Itching or aching	Hay fever
Eyes	Itching, burning, or tearing	Hay fever, allergic conjunctivitis
Mouth and throat	Swelling of mucus tissue	Food allergy, insect stings or bites
Circulatory (vascular) system	Low blood pressure, faintness	Anaphylaxis Food allergy

*The symptoms listed are *possibly* the result of allergic disease. However, all of them can be brought on by nonallergic conditions. The mere presence of the symptoms should not be taken as incontrovertible evidence that an allergy is to blame.

**Only the most common allergic diseases are represented in the table.

lergy Finder (Figure 1). If your youngster is troubled with symptoms that might be due to an allergy, you can use the Finder to narrow down the possible causes, and at the same time, be somewhat more confident about knowing what is causing the symptoms. Carefully maintaining the Allergy Finder and taking it along to your doctor will help in deciding whether or not your child's problems are due to an allergy.

DIRECTIONS FOR USING THE ALLERGY FINDER

Fill out the Allergy Finder each evening, just before the child goes to bed. It should take you only a few minutes. For the SYMPTOMS section, if the child had no symptoms that day, leave the spaces blank; if there were symptoms, indicate what they were (sneezing; runny nose; wheezing; coughing; upset stomach; nausea; diarrhea; etc.) and when they appeared, how severe they were, and whether or not they disappeared or persisted and got worse.

For all other sections, check every item for which you have a "yes"

TABLE 3
Allergic Diseases and Their Characteristics

ALLERGIC DISEASE	*USUAL AGE OF ONSET*	*APPEARANCE AND PROGRESS OF SYMPTOMS*
Eczema	6 months or older	Starts with intense itching accompanied by scratching, restlessness, sleep disturbance; lesions then appear, their character and location dependent on child's age and degree of severity
Hives	Uncommon before 2 years	Sudden appearance of wheals (slightly raised inflamed areas), followed by intense itching; wheals usually disappear within a few hours but may migrate to other parts of body
Seasonal hay fever	4–18 years	Repetitive sneezing with itching of palate, throat, and ear canal; usually seasonal, particularly springtime, and made worse on high-pollen-count and windy days
Chronic hay fever	4–18 years	Repetitive year-round sneezing, often worse indoors and when exposed to dust. Sneezing with throat, palate, and ear canal itching; often associated with clogged ears and sinusitis
Asthma	18 months to any age	Shortness of breath, coughing, wheezing
Food allergy	Birth to any age	Diarrhea, colic; can involve almost any organ or system in the body, triggering hay fever, hives, eczema, or asthma

answer that day. In the FOODS section make a special effort to record everything that the child ate.

To interpret the form, at the end of the week count the number of check marks that you have made for each entry and record the number in the "Total" column at the right. Then relate the entries in the SYMPTOMS section to those in all of the other sections: For example, if you checked no symptoms all week, what other categories or items had no check that week? If the child did have symptoms, which of the other boxes were also checked on the day before or on the day the symptoms showed? If the child was troubled with symptoms throughout the whole week, which boxes had checks every day? Write any suspected matchup of symptoms and causes on a sheet of paper as illustrated below:

Dates	*Symptoms*	*Possible Causes*
______	______	______
______	______	______
______	______	______
______	______	______
______	______	______

FIGURE 1 Allergy Finder

For ______________________ (Name) Week of ______________________ (Month) to ______________________ (Dates) 19____

	Mon	Tue	Wed	Thu	Fri	Sat	Sun	Total
WHAT WERE THE SYMPTOMS?								
WHEN DID THE SYMPTOMS SHOW?								
Morning								
Afternoon								
Evening								
During the night								
HOW SEVERE WERE THE SYMPTOMS?								
No symptoms seen								
Mild								
Moderate								
Severe								
DID THE SYMPTOMS								
Disappear?								
Disappear and return?								
Persist?								
Persist and worsen?								
WAS THE WEATHER								
Cold?								
Snowy/Rainy?								
Windy?								
Hot/Humid?								

FIGURE 1 Allergy Finder (continued)

	Mon	Tue	Wed	Thu	Fri	Sat	Sun	Total
DID THE CHILD HAVE ANY INFECTIONS?								
Cold								
Flu								
Sinusitis								
Other*								
WHERE DID THE CHILD GO? WHAT DID HE OR SHE DO?								
Day care								
Preschool								
School								
Home								
Work								
Travel/Dine out/Recreation								
Played outside								
Exercised vigorously								
Other*								
WAS THE CHILD EXPOSED TO								
Smoke/Tobacco?								
Dust/Pollen?								
Mold/Dampness?								
Auto emissions?								
Other fumes?								
Animals/Pets?								
Chemicals or solvents?								
Other airborne irritants?*								
DID THE CHILD USE, WEAR, OR COME IN CONTACT WITH								
Cigarettes?								
Detergents/Soaps?								
Perfume/Cosmetics?								
Bath preparations?								
Wool/Fur/Leather?								
Jewelry?								
Poison oak, ivy, sumac?								
Insecticides or other chemicals?								
Other suspected triggers?*								

* Specify

FIGURE 1 Allergy Finder (continued)

	Mon	Tue	Wed	Thu	Fri	Sat	Sun	Total
DID THE CHILD TAKE ANY DRUGS OR MEDICATIONS? Aspirin								
Other pain or headache remedy*								
Cold medicine*								
Nose drops*								
Skin medication*								
Antibiotics*								
Other*								
DID THE CHILD EXPERIENCE ANY UNUSUAL STRESS, TENSION, ANXIETY, OR CONFLICT?								
WHAT DID THE CHILD EAT? Grains or cereals (breads, pastries, breakfast foods)								
Milk or milk products (ice cream, cheese, sour cream, cottage cheese, yogurt, etc.)								
Eggs/egg products								
Poultry								
Meats (fresh or processed)								
Fish or shellfish								
Raw fruits or vegetables								
Snacks, including candies								
Chocolate								
Nuts or nut butter								
Popcorn								
Chewing gum								
Beverages, including tea								
coffee								
cola/soda								
beer, wine, or other alcohol								

*Specify

It may be necessary to keep the Allergy Finder for a number of weeks, so we encourage you to photocopy it beforehand.

THE DOCTOR'S ROLE

For confident diagnosis of allergy in your child and prescription of appropriate remedies you need to see your doctor. Chapter 22 tells you how to go about choosing a physician and describes the procedures he or she will observe in treating your youngster. In summary, here are the steps your doctor will follow:

1. A good, detailed history.
2. A complete, thorough physical examination that includes measures of height, weight, blood pressure, inspection of ears, nose, eyes, mouth, throat, listening to heart and lungs, and close examination of skin plus information on general health practices, diet, sleep, exercise, etc.

   (These first two steps, carefully carried out, are often enough to provide a firm diagnosis. If they do not, then some of the following tests may be required.)

3. Skin (called scratch, prick, or intradermal) tests done in the doctor's office to detect sensitivity to substances possibly causing the allergic reaction. (Skin tests should be used with caution; they are not appropriate for young children or if eczema is present or for any child who is having an allergic flare-up or asthma attack at the time of testing.)
4. Laboratory blood tests (called RAST or FAST) that determine the presence of heightened levels of immunoglobulin E. These tests can confirm that an IgE or allergic antibody is present but do not pin down the cause any better than skin tests.
5. Challenge tests, usually done in hospital or clinic. These tests directly assess the reaction to suspected allergens. They entail some risks, are not appropriate for all allergic reactions, and should be considered a last resort.

ALLERGIES AND ALLERGY IMPOSTERS

Allergies unfairly catch the blame for too many complaints. "I think he's allergic to something," a parent may say to explain a child's skin irritation, chronic runny nose, intestinal upset, headache, or virtually any other ailment the body is subject to.

There are a number of good reasons for this unfortunate tendency toward indiscriminate labeling. "Allergy" has gradually taken on a meaning much broader than its original one. You have doubtless heard, seen, or perhaps even lightheartedly made statements like these: "I'm allergic to my boss," "my teacher," "my in-laws," "math," "Christmas." In this context you declare yourself "allergic" to any source of discomfort, annoyance, or frustration, and you may also diagnose "allergy" when troubled with any symptom or condition whose cause is unknown to you.

Lucy chain smokes. Whenever she smokes her six-year-old son Eric begins coughing. She is convinced that Eric is allergic to smoke. Totally addicted, she can't give up cigarettes, and Eric can't seem to stop coughing. In desperation she turns to an allergist hoping that Eric will be able to get allergy shots to help his condition. The allergist patiently tries to explain that Eric is not allergic to the smoke. It is merely an irritant that is noxious for his lungs. Lucy can't seem to understand. "I know he is allergic to smoke," she says. "I know, because he coughs when I smoke."

Doctors have also contributed to the terminological muddle. They have used the word loosely, sometimes calling a reaction allergic when it is really due to something else they consider too difficult or involved to explain to the patient.

Then there is the scenario that goes like this: Your child has a recurring problem — for instance, diarrhea, or constipation, a skin rash, a chronic runny nose, ear infections. You take the child to the doctor, who may run a diagnostic test. The test is inconclusive. "Probably an allergy," the doctor says and sends you to a specialist who orders more tests, finds nothing clear-cut, and also declares that the symptoms are due to an allergic reaction for which treatment, which may or may not work, is prescribed. In instances like these "allergy" becomes a diagnostic wastebasket into which unexplained symptoms are dumped. Or the word may refer to symptoms that look as if they ought to be allergic reactions but are really attributable to an allergy imposter.

Dr. Paul is one of those wonderful old-fashioned general practitioners. Over the years he has learned that he doesn't have everything to offer all patients, but he has always felt obliged to tell his patients what the trouble is — to give them a diagnosis. One of his patients is Jackie, a teenager. Jackie is chronically constipated and very troubled and embarrassed by it. The good doctor checked her carefully, recommended that she take a glass of prune juice each morning, and added by way of explanation and reassurance, "Jackie, you're probably just allergic to certain foods." Unfortunately, while the prune juice treatment worked just fine, Jackie became concerned about the ill-considered suggestion that her problem was rooted in an allergy. She went on a protracted, exhaustive food elimination diet that proved totally uninformative; she and her parents spent almost $100 on a useless collection of books on food allergies and allergic diets; and she developed a phobia about foods that persists to this day. The doctor's careless, unreflective attribution of the problem to "allergy" played havoc with Jackie.

Allergic reactions are expressed in a limited number of symptoms — the most common ones are named and discussed in Part III. Most of these symptoms can also be allergy imposters; that is, they can be the outcome of nonallergic reactions. For example, suppose your two-year-old is subject to frequent ear infections. The principal reason for ear infections in young children is blockage, inflammation, and infection in the eustachian tube. The eustachian tube is a pipe that links the nose to the ear drum; if the tube becomes inflamed, as is often the case during a cold, normal drainage is hindered. Waste builds up, bacteria invade and multiply, and an ear infection develops. In this instance the symptoms are allergy imposters.

Exactly the same symptoms can be caused by a eustachian tube closed by hay fever, an allergic condition that can and often does trigger a chain of events identical to those associated with a cold.

It may not seem all that important to make the distinction between earaches due to allergy and those caused by an allergy imposter. The pain, the crying, the distress, and the treatment for the condition are the same regardless of cause. Yet, knowing the underlying reason is crucial because, with that knowledge, the parent is helped to forestall possible future episodes and to deal with them efficiently and intelligently if they do recur.

ALLERGY, ALLERGY IMPOSTERS, AND PHYSIOLOGY

As it happens, the physical changes that children experience as they pass through the stages from newborn baby to adolescent are implicated in the allergy — imposter confusion.

- Earaches become less frequent and severe as the child matures and the eustachian tube enlarges.
- Colic or gastric upsets gradually disappear as the digestive system matures to the point where it can handle milk efficiently.
- Episodes of wheezing and asthma tend to become less severe or vanish altogether as the airways in the respiratory system enlarge.

Thus, many childhood symptoms — whether allergy-caused or simply allergylike — moderate or disappear as the physical development of the child proceeds or as the immunological system matures. (Infants are apt to have 10 or more colds a year; the figure drops to 4 or 5 in primary school youngsters. Exposure and repeated infection help build resistance.)

3.

Guiding Your Allergic Child into the Mainstream

We designed this book to help parents recognize, manage, and prevent their children's allergic problems. Much of what we discuss concerns avoiding allergen contact or exposure *at home*. However, as every parent realizes, a child's universe begins expanding from the day of birth, continually widening with exposure to different environments, new situations, changed responsibilities. During their formative years children spend many hours in school or at the homes of friends; those with working parents have lengthy periods of time at home alone; they may celebrate holidays or special occasions more actively than adults do; they attend summer camp, travel, or vacation with their families. For the allergic child, each of these aspects of growing up represents a special circumstance and poses certain risks — risks that can be met and countered with careful planning and forethought.

GENERAL HEALTH PROBLEMS

While there are any number of problems that can grow out of allergic conditions, the most common and troublesome ones are associated with either the child's general health or his or her school performance. General health problems arising out of allergic conditions occur often enough to be a matter of concern to parents. These can range from chronic eye or ear problems to low energy level or little resistance to recurring infections like colds and flu or chronic ones like sinusitis. Here are some of the things parents can do to deal effectively with the possibility that an allergy has in some way undermined the child's general health:

1. Monitor the child's behavior to the extent that you can become aware of any substantial departures from the ordinary — lassitude, apathy, hyperactivity, change in sleep patterns or needs, complaints about not feeling well, stomachache, headache, and so forth. (Try to keep your eye on the child without becoming obsessive or oversolicitous about it; these are mistakes that carry their own separate recipes for disaster.)
2. If the atypical behavior persists for more than a day or two, talk openly and matter-of-factly with the youngster about it. If necessary, check the child's temperature, breathing, and so on.
3. Be alert to the fact that some allergy medications can produce the symptoms named above. Review the child's medications and find out their possible side effects.
4. Confer with your doctor, describing the symptoms fully (onset, nature, severity, what you have done about them), and request and act on the doctor's recommendations.

SCHOOL PROBLEMS

Depending on the allergy or allergies, life at school can present serious complications to the families of allergic children. The nature of your child's allergies — asthma, eczema, hay fever — will have you thinking about whether or not he or she should use the cafeteria, take physical education, go on field trips, and attend school or class parties. You will wonder about the advisability of taking certain subjects, the degree of contact with other children, and so on. To deal with these questions effectively you and your child need to know as much as possible about the causes of and the methods of controlling allergies. Here are some questions you should consider, have the answers to, and discuss with school authorities (principal, teachers, counselor, nurse) before school begins.

1. Do your child's allergies appear during or get worse with exercise?
2. Do sharp or pungent odors trigger or intensify your child's allergies?
3. Does ordinary soap cause skin irritation or eczema in your child?
4. Does your child have food allergies?
5. Does exposure to heat or dust make your child's allergies get worse?
6. Does handling clay, glue, or other substances cause contact allergies (dermatitis) in your child?
7. Does your child feel troubled or conspicuous at being left out of certain programs or activities?

8. Do you, the child, and school officials know what to do about the foregoing problems?
9. Do you know the school policy about administering medication during the school day? Have you worked out a mutually satisfactory and thoroughly understood procedure for getting medication to the child when it is needed?
10. Do you, the school, and the child know what to do if the child develops symptoms at school? Have you agreed on a procedure to follow if symptoms intensify or become serious? What is the school's policy for managing medical emergencies?

Overall School Performance

Allergies, especially hay fever and asthma, can pull down school performance, either directly by forcing frequent, extended absences or indirectly by requiring medication that makes the child hyperactive or drowsy and inattentive. Get to know your child's abilities and level of performance through your own observations, consultation with teachers and counselor, and familiarity with the past academic record. If performance starts sliding, talk with the child and the teacher or teachers involved. Concentrate on finding out what is happening and why. Asking the child (and teachers) to describe specific events or behavior will probably lead to some hunches about the reasons for the falloff. Where the problem is associated with activity-type subjects requiring physical activity (physical education particularly), try to establish the nature of the difficulty and, in cooperation with child and teacher, work out a solution that everyone can live with.

Help the child by trying to determine the real reason for the poor performance and getting rid of it. Scrupulously avoid doing the work for the child. That will do nothing at all to solve whatever academic difficulties he or she is having and is a poor precedent to set for later difficulties, should they occur.

Physical Education

Physical education is an important part of the school program. While there are some children who have physical disabilities that make it impossible for them to participate in such programs, this is *not* the case for children with allergies. Youngsters with hay fever, eczema, or even asthma may participate in physical education provided commonsense precautions and limitations are observed. First, if your child has eczema and washes or showers after exercise, it is important to avoid all soaps without fail or use nonsoap skin cleansers. Children are often very self-conscious about not using soap in a communal situation and, to avoid teasing and embarrassment, may soap up like the rest of the kids. The child should be helped by you and the teacher not to give in to this sort of pressure.

Andy has had eczema for as long as he can remember. While most boys hate baths, Andy has come to resent his mother's harping about avoiding soap. He is now 13 and on the school basketball team. His eczema has been pretty well controlled for years. However, in the shower, when all the team members lathered themselves with soap suds, Andy joined in the fun. Three days later his skin was painfully red and dry. A day after that the skin started to crack and small localized infections started. Finally Andy could stand it no longer and showed the sores to his mom. She packed him off to their dermatologist, who prescribed a heavy treatment of steroid creams and delivered an even heavier lecture to Andy.

Children with hay fever can exercise and play with the same intensity as any other children. Children receiving good medical treatment for their hay fever should have no problems whatsoever; but if your child is in the throes of a hay fever attack, it is best that he or she stay quiet and indoors, off the playground, or out of the gym until medication has the symptoms under firm control.

Antihistamines, which are frequently prescribed for mild cases of hay fever, may make children sleepy, adversely affect school performance, and interfere with attentiveness at school. The school should know if your child is on antihistamines; we discuss this issue at length in Chapter 12. We do not recommend drugs that cause sedation in children!

Children with asthma are in by far the worst situation. Even mild exercise may trigger some degree of wheezing in virtually every asthmatic child. This should be forestalled; often judicious use of medication before exercise will fend off symptoms. If your child starts to wheeze or wheezes more severely during exercise, it is prudent he or she avoid hard physical exertion. Redirection into exercises or activities that are more appropriate for asthmatic children would be helpful; swimming is, by far, the most suitable. Most middle and high schools of any size offer "adaptive" physical education activities for children unable to do the regular program comfortably. Your child should get advice from the doctor about steps to take to prevent exercise-induced asthma.

Other Classes

We believe that children with allergies should be given the opportunity to take the full spectrum of courses and that their academic choices should not be limited because of their illness. Fortunately, for the majority of allergic children this is not an issue. The appropriate and timely use of medication effectively prevents symptoms from developing.

Some strong, pungent fumes or odors can trigger asthma or other allergies. This usually occurs in high school and college chemistry labs where fumes can be strong enough to bring on wheezing. The villains here are mainly sulfur dioxide or hydrogen sulfide, which smell like rotten eggs. A paper mask is sometimes all it takes to prevent reactions; in other instances a more aggressive medication program may be necessary. All asthmatic children should be wary of chemistry laboratories.

> Anne did so well in math and science that she was accepted for a special National Science Foundation program for bright high school kids at the University of California at Berkeley. During her first week of classes she was assigned to work in an organic chemistry lab. Although most of the chemistry took place under special hoods where the gases are sucked away and dispersed outside, the lab still smelled of acids and ethers, esters, and sulfur. Anne, who had suffered from asthma during childhood, suddenly found herself coughing during each chemistry lab. While it was only a cough she was uncomfortable and did feel her chest getting tight. She did not think it was asthma because she remembered hearing herself wheeze as a child and there were no wheezes this time. Nonetheless, she went to the Student Health Center where the doctor listened to her with a stethoscope. His first question was, "Have you ever been told you have asthma?" Anne couldn't believe her ears. She had not had a wheeze in over six years. They discussed the situation and the fact that the cough seemed to get worse in the chemistry lab. The doctor suggested a special mask. Anne used it and had no problems thereafter.

Contact with a wide range of substances at school can also trigger allergic symptoms. In younger children, paints, pastes, glues, or modeling clay can and often do bring on contact dermatitis. In older children classes in art, shop, and cooking expose them to unusual dusts (wood, flour) and fumes (solder flux, glue, paint). Cleaning solutions and a variety of other materials can bring on dermatitis as well as nasal or respiratory problems. Excessive heat can intensify eczema; dust from sweeping, chalkboard, playground, or heating vents can provoke hay fever or asthma; air conditioning units can spew asthma- or hay fever-causing mold into the environment. Anything at all that causes allergies at home can turn up at school. In addition, there is more opportunity at school for the transmission of colds and respiratory infections.

The possible causes of allergies and methods of avoiding them are covered in Part II. Your job, as parent, is to be alert to the appearance of symptoms and to review your child's activities carefully. (*This may well be the hardest part of your job*! Most children are infuriatingly laconic when asked to talk about their activities.) Pin down the cause of the reaction, and then take action to treat the symptoms and, in cooperation with the school, remove or avoid their cause or causes.

Other Risks at School

For children with serious food hypersensitivities, the school lunch can be a problem. Sometimes it is hard to know what is in school cafeteria food. If your child reacts to some common foods like flour, peanut butter, and milk, pack an appropriate lunch and send it along to school with the youngster, or instruct the child to prepare the proper foods without your help.

Perhaps the more serious problem, though, is the intense peer pressure not to be different. This is reflected in the extraordinary and sometimes dangerous lengths kids will go to in order to seem just like everybody else. In teenaged girls, for instance, there has recently been an enormous increase in the use of beauty aids — face and eye makeup, shampoos, scents, fingernail preparations. In girls with eczema or contact dermatitis, makeup can provoke or aggravate skin problems tragically.

For both boys and girls there is pressure to drink alcohol, to smoke or dip snuff, and to wear certain kinds of clothes. The first two habits are illegal as well as dangerous for any child; for allergic children they can be exceptionally hazardous — in some instances lethal. And in certain allergic youngsters even wearing the "right" kinds of clothes — rubber, wool, plastics, leather — can bring on troublesome skin reactions.

Here you, the parent, have to remind the child of his or her uniqueness and vulnerability and the need to take appropriate precautions. Worse, you have to do it without pushing the child into rebellion, withdrawal, or overdependence on you.

PROBLEMS AT HOME AND AWAY

At Homes of Friends

When an allergic child visits or sleeps over at a friend's house both the child and the parent or parents of the friend need to know how to deal with any problems that may erupt. You should see to it that your child carries along whatever is needed to avoid or manage difficulties encountered at the friend's house, including medications and any special preparations or equipment required for allergy treatment. The friend's parents should be aware (beforehand) of the allergy, how it manifests itself, and what triggers it — foods, exercise, pets — and what to do if anything happens. Your child can help by behaving responsibly in this unfamiliar environment.

At Home Alone

Millions of children are "latchkey kids," returning to an empty home while parent or parents are away at work. In addition to the routine precautions and communication strategies that this situation demands, allergic latchkey kids have to be responsible for watching out for their allergies. They should know what they must do to avoid or control triggers, when, how, and how much to medicate, and what activities are permissible. Allergic children live in a world with limits. Your job is to teach them what these boundaries are. Small contributions on your part can help greatly; for example, if your child has food allergies, preparing the ritual after-school snack beforehand and leaving it in a special place in the refrigerator will guard against your child's eating something that may bring on wheezing, hives, stomach upset, or any of the other symptoms that food allergy produces.

Where substantial risk to the child is involved — shock reactions to foods, insect stings, severe wheezing brought on by exertion or infection, and so on — you need to take two additional precautions. First, recruit someone dependable like a neighbor or nearby relative who is willing and trained (by you) to know exactly what to do and who can minister to the child in an emergency. Instruct the child to call this emergency care provider if anything goes wrong. Second, arrange it so that people know where and how you can be reached at work if that should become necessary. Have a written procedures list they can follow for allergic emergencies.

Holidays

Holidays are risky times for any child. In addition to overdosing on food, activity, and excitement, children are likely to encounter different foods in unfamiliar settings. For allergic youngsters the risks are even greater.

> Randy, an eight-year-old, has had asthma since he was two. His mother has noticed that he always get worse right around Christmas. The doctor suggested that he might be allergic to the Christmas tree. In fact, one year they had an outdoor Christmas tree and Randy was better during that season,

although he continued to wheeze somewhat. The doctor also asked about unusual activities restricted to the season. "We keep a fire going in the fireplace and we use a lot of candles, scented ones," Randy's mom said. "Cut them out next time and see what happens," the doctor advised. It wasn't like their traditional Christmas: no tree, no cheerful fire crackling in the fireplace, no candles. No asthma either.

In most instances, if you know what triggers your child's allergies, and what you and your child must do to avoid and treat them, you can get through any holiday by being watchful and imposing and enforcing whatever allergy-dodging steps are necessary. This may put a mild damper on the festivities, but a safe and sane celebration is clearly to be preferred to one where flaring allergies ruin everyone's fun.

Traveling

Travel, particularly the kind that involves staying in strange places or eating out-of-the-ordinary foods or engaging in unaccustomed activities, can be accompanied by the development of symptoms. If you have an allergic child, *never* leave home on a trip without carrying an adequate supply of medicine.

As far as accommodations are concerned, depending on the allergy and its trigger, you may want to look for places to stay that do not admit pets, that offer tobacco-free rooms, or that on inspection seem to be clean and mold-free. Ask to look at the room first. If the trigger is not the kind you can spot, ask the innkeeper the relevant questions.

Lew, 10, has an acute hypersensitivity reaction to perfumed fabric softeners, the strips of chemically treated paper thrown into a clothes dryer to make the wash soft and "fragrant." Whenever he touches anything that has been in contact with one of these chemicals — sheets, pillowcases, towels, clothing — he breaks out with a severe case of hives. From bitter experience Lew's parents have learned to ask first if the motel uses fabric softeners on the sheets and towels. If the answer is "Yes" or "Don't know" then find another place.

Strange foods (or additives) can also cause problems to the unwary. To an extent they can be avoided if you do what you can (and you can do a lot) to supply your own food as you go. However, if your family's mode of travel entails driving day and night straight through, stopping only to refuel or to get food at a fast-food place, expect problems.

What is true of public accommodations is also true of public transportation. Buses, planes, and trains are generally inadequately ventilated and may be contaminated with pollutants. If this is the case, complain. You are entitled to clean air to breathe.

Note, also, that federal and state regulations prohibit smoking on some airline flights; a few carriers have outlawed it altogether. If necessary, seek out and patronize these health-conscious firms. And, if a complaint becomes necessary, take it to the highest level, the president or chief executive officer of the company. It won't help your child this trip, but long-run policy changes may result.

The food on board or in the terminals or depots is likely to have been prepared well in advance, and laced with salt and preservatives. It is possible if traveling by air to order special vegetarian or kosher meals beforehand; but there are no special provisions for the allergic traveler, whose only recourse is to beware.

Summer Camp

Summer camp is a memorable experience in any case; it is particularly worthwhile for children with allergies, especially asthma. Many years ago a Denver-based group began a summer camp called Camp Broncho, to "buck" asthma; they called the campers "bucking bronchos." This was a daring and innovative move at the time; since then respiratory societies and lung associations all over America have promoted the use of summer camps for children with asthma. They are usually attended by physicians who volunteer their time. Nursing supervision is also provided so that the children are monitored and keep up with their medicine. The camps are extraordinarily helpful for several reasons:

1. Camps give parents time away from their chronically asthmatic children.
2. Asthmatic children meet and learn from one another.
3. Children develop self-esteem and a sense of competency, control over their disease, and self-worth.
4. Camps provide sound, protective, fun-filled environments.

Appendix G lists, by state, organizations that sponsor such summer programs. If none of these is in your area, ask your local American Lung Association branch for names and addresses of nearby camps.

SPECIAL PROBLEMS OF ALLERGIC CHILDREN

Allergic kids are like other children. They need to and can be treated like other youngsters without people making a great to-do over their condition. They experience all of the events of growing up other children do and, for the most part, need neither shielding nor special help. There are a few things, however, that sometimes roughen the path a bit; these possible complications are covered in this section. Later we deal with the special significance that headaches (Chapter 18), fever (Chapter 19), and colds (Chapter 20) hold for allergic youngsters.

Injuries (cuts and lacerations, sprains, fractures) are a routine feature of growing up. They themselves do not represent an added hazard to allergic children, but their treatment can sometimes precipitate problems. Depending on the severity of the injury, it may be necessary to prescribe pain relievers or antibiotics (to guard against infection) or to give a tetanus booster.

Antipain medication, anything that contains aspirin or codeine, should be administered cautiously to allergic kids. It should absolutely not be given to asthmatics where the drug can either trigger the reaction (aspirin) or depress the respiratory system (codeine). Tetanus shots do not in themselves carry any threat to allergic children, but if the child dreads the needle, the fear can sometimes affect the breathing and intensify respiratory problems.

Antibiotics, especially penicillin, are notorious triggers of allergic reactions. They should be administered only if the need for them is clear and then only if the physician knows that your child has allergies.

Fungus infections, especially of feet and hands, are a routine nuisance in children. For the most part, they can be managed readily by careful washing and by keeping the affected areas dry and open to the air as much as possible. Fungus infections (and some of the many over-the-counter medications available for the treatment of athlete's foot, jock itch, and other variations on fungus infections) sometimes interact with existing skin allergies, notably eczema and allergic contact dermatitis, and need to be treated carefully and as conservatively as possible.

Skin eruptions, pimples and acne, are a matter of great concern to many adolescents. For the most part, these blemishes are self-limiting, clearing up on their own in time. There is a huge arsenal of topical medications around to treat these conditions, some of them fairly effective, most of them without merit. However, the treatments (and the alternative tactic of covering the sores with makeup) can cause hypersensitivity or allergic reactions (triggering allergic contact dermatitis; worsening eczema) and probably ought to be avoided by teenagers with allergy-related skin problems.

Dental problems are the bane of everyone's existence. Allergic kids are going to need to have their teeth cleaned, cavities filled, and, in some instances, extractions made and orthodontic work carried out. Where dental work is concerned, there are a few things that parents of allergic kids should be alert to. The anesthetics used to block pain (novocaine or other "caines") can trigger hives or more serious shock reactions in some susceptible individuals; postoperative pain remedies (as with *injuries*) may also cause difficulties.

Drugs and alcohol are bad news for anyone, but they carry an added threat for allergic children. Alcohol and some recreational drugs can greatly compromise the respiratory and vascular systems and so represent a real danger to asthmatics especially.

OTHER PROBLEMS

In addition to the special problems and risks that ordinary diseases or conditions may represent to allergic kids, there is the hard fact that some must be denied certain kinds of experiences other children are free to enjoy. Prominent among these is the freedom to have and enjoy pets. For children who react to respiratory allergens, the plea to keep a dog or cat or horse or bird should be denied, kindly but firmly and with a sympathetic explanation. Where a pet is already on the scene and causing problems, find it a good foster home; this can be a bitter pill to take, especially for children who are strongly attached to their pets. However, keeping it would only bring you and your child a different kind of grief.

It may also be necessary to exercise a lot of care in choosing the kinds of toys an allergic youngster has. For kids with respiratory allergies, soft, cuddly dolls — dust-catching teddy bears, giant pandas, and other plush playmates especially — may have to be returned to the wild. This may cause a crisis, but it will pass. Misunderstanding and disappointment can be avoided if giftgivers (grandparents, especially) are told ahead of time what toys and gifts are appropriate — and inappropriate — for the allergic child.

TEACHING ALLERGIC OFFSPRING HOW TO ACT JUDICIOUSLY AND COMPETENTLY ON THEIR OWN

It has been found that even very young children — four- and five-year-olds — can, with proper coaching, learn to manage their own allergies competently. This is especially true for asthmatic children — so true, in fact, that there are a number of brief self-management programs that have been developed especially to help asthmatic children deal with their symptoms. Your local lung association branch or HMO will know of these offerings. Children who have other kinds of allergies do not have the advantage of being able to participate in such ready-made programs. Nonetheless, parents can do an effective job of teaching their children how to manage their allergic symptoms. In doing this there are several important precepts you must keep in mind.

First, the child has to know exactly what the allergy is, what triggers it, and what to do to avoid the reaction. *Second*, the parents and other health care providers must spend the time and energy to convey the avoidance and treatment strategies in terms the child can comprehend. Then, present a situation in which the child might realistically find himself or herself (or has already been) and ask, "What are the things you should do?" Repetition and positive reinforcement ("That's fine!" "Exactly right!") will ensure the success of this phase of the learning program.

Third, parents and health care providers must show children how to go about making their own independent health care decisions, give them the freedom and opportunity to do so, and review the decisions and their outcomes carefully. This is probably the most difficult step of all for parents. Not wanting to put the child at risk, parents are inclined to make these sorts of decisions themselves without consulting the child. Worse still, they strive to create an environment altogether free of hazards. This oversolicitude and lack of confidence in the capacity of the child to act intelligently in his or her own behalf tends to foster long-term and sometimes crippling dependence on the parents. It certainly interferes with the child's need to be self-reliant.

Most childhood allergies ease up or disappear during the process of growing up. Where the allergic condition is chronic and persistent, medications and other preventive or avoidance tactics can usually hold the symptoms in check. In short, where parent and child are informed, alert, and thoughtful, allergic children, even those moderately to severely troubled, can and should be helped and encouraged to do the sorts of things nonallergic youngsters do. The suggestions we have outlined here are designed to help parents help their allergic kids to venture into the mainstream of youthful life safely and enjoyably.

PART TWO

WHAT ARE ALLERGIES' TRIGGERS AND HOW CAN I AVOID OR CONTROL THEM EFFECTIVELY?

4.

Food and Food Additives

Almost everyone has at one time or another had a reaction that they choose to call a food allergy. This near-universal claim needs to be scrutinized more closely. Take the word "food." Food is not only the name of whatever is eaten but actually all of the materials used to prepare, preserve, and color it, plus the residue from packaging or storage materials and contaminants like pesticides, herbicides, and insect or rodent leavings and remains.

Identifying and then dealing with food allergies or intolerances is one of the more complex and difficult areas in the whole field of allergy. This chapter simply identifies some of the more common causes of these food-linked symptoms, tells how they are expressed, and discusses the symptoms, diagnosis, and treatment of these conditions.

A food *allergy* is an immune-mediated reaction by the body against the foodstuff itself or something else contained in it. (See Chapter 1 for more on the nature of an allergy.)

Actually, what is popularly called a food allergy is in almost all cases an "intolerance," a local irritant effect like the heartburn from spicy foods, a headache from too much wine, or diarrhea from too many prunes. Perhaps 1% of all reactions to foods are true allergies; the rest are intolerances, reactions to something consumed that did not agree with us or carried distressing side effects.

Most true allergic reactions to food are found in children. As with other allergies, there is an anatomical reason for this. Food is introduced into the mouth in either liquid or semiliquid form or is so rendered by the process of chewing. It then passes along to the stomach and intestine where digestion takes place; that is, the material is broken down into subunits or very "short" chemicals. These "short" chemicals are then absorbed into the body tissues where they fuel our cells. In infants and toddlers the intestines are immature, not yet completely developed. Digestion is incomplete, permitting the absorption of "larger" chemicals or actual bits of the food itself into the body. These "larger" chemicals from food are seen by the body's immune system as invaders, and the immune response is triggered.

Milk offers a good example of how all this happens. When adults drink milk its principal proteins are rapidly broken down by the stomach leaving only the "short" chemicals; in children minute quantities of the whole, undigested proteins can sometimes be detected in the blood.

SYMPTOMS OF FOOD ALLERGY OR INTOLERANCE

Food (or whatever else food contains) can affect almost any organ or system of the body, and so the symptoms of food allergy can take an astonishing variety of forms. Some of them bear what seems like little or no rational connection to their original cause.

Gastrointestinal symptoms are the most frequent result of food intolerance in young children; but symptoms can also be expressed as skin disorders either directly (triggering hives and rashes) or indirectly (making eczema worse); as respiratory problems, especially wheezing and shortness of breath; as vascular complications ranging from mild headache to sudden, catastrophic drop in blood pressure; as itching and swelling of mucus tissue, especially of the throat (palate) or lips; and as abdominal pain. Onset can be sudden or gradual and not necessarily limited to one organ or area; hives and wheezing and/or vascular problems often occur together. Symptoms can be short-lived, vanishing in an hour or two, or they can persist for days as prolonged and acute distress. In short, when taken together, adverse reactions to food can add up to a very complex maze of symptoms.

DIAGNOSTIC PROCEDURES FOR ESTABLISHING THE CAUSE OF FOOD ALLERGIES OR INTOLERANCES

Because of the variety of symptoms and their unpredictable onset and course, establishing the cause for food intolerances is difficult. At the University of California, Davis, Medical Center about 20% of all new patients at the Allergy and Immunology Clinic complain of a food allergy. In a handful of these individuals, the causal connection between trigger and symptom is obvious; the time between ingestion of the offending food and appearance of symptoms is measured in minutes. In the remaining 80% of cases, however, the history of the problem is confusing and the cause unclear or uncertain with physician and patient having little to go on to establish a clear-cut diagnosis.

Bobby, 11, was referred to the clinic because of a puzzling history of recurring hives. Approximately three times a year, without warning, Bobby would break out with severe, itchy hives all over his body. He and his parents are absolutely convinced that food is responsible. Because the episodes occur irregularly, Bobby's recollection of what he has eaten is not particularly dependable, and he is often unable to remember having eaten anything unusual. While there is no clear link between his hives and some specific food consumed, his parents and he stubbornly hold to the view that food is doing the damage.

The doctors who examined Bobby are in a dilemma. They know he has hives because they can see the wheals all over his body. Yet, because the hives turn up so irregularly and are not accompanied by any obvious inciting factors, the doctors are in the dark as to the causes. Bobby and his parents want the clinic to run skin tests to nail down the food that is responsible for his troubles. They refuse to accept the argument that there are no reliable, accurate ways of testing for Bobby's alleged food allergy. Yet, there are a number of reasons why this statement is true.

Food is such a complex mix of materials and undergoes so many chemical changes during its production, preservation, storage, preparation, and digestion that tens of thousands of combinations of what represents the substance to be tested are possible. The skin test, discussed in Chapter 12, is the mainstay for identifying respiratory allergens, but it is not especially effective when it comes to identifying food allergens. (Most allergists will not order skin tests for food allergies or insensitivities; the ones who do do so with great misgivings and have little hope that the tests will point to a single clear-cut cause.)

There are other kinds of tests to determine if an allergic reaction is present in the body when symptoms show. For example, blood tests, called RAST or FAST, are not designed to pin down the cause of a reaction; they simply indicate whether the reaction, whatever it is, has produced IgE antibodies. These tests also yield unpredictable and sometimes confusing results. In small children, for example, researchers have found IgE antibodies not only in children allergic to milk but in those who do not have a milk allergy. Worse, they have detected no antibodies in children who have what seems to be a clear-cut history of milk allergy.

Some physicians also offer cytotoxic or sublingual (under the tongue) tests. Cytotoxic testing, a laboratory procedure that purports to analyze the effects of suspected food on white blood cells, has been studied carefully and found to be devoid of any scientific merit; sublingual testing has also been the subject of several extensive reviews that question the procedure's utility. If your doctor recommends such testing we recommend that you consult another physician to get a second opinion.

To discover what food or foods are causing a reaction in your child, an *elimination diet* can help you. What such a diet does is to start out by limiting the child to a few foods that are almost never responsible for reactions. Then, at regular intervals, additional foods are added and the reactions of the child to them are observed carefully. If the child shows a reaction the food suspected of causing it is dropped from the diet and then reintroduced after a waiting period. If the reaction occurs after the second exposure, there is good reason to believe that the offending food has been found. A general elimination diet is given in Appendix A. Specific diets free of mold, tyramine, salicylate, cereals, and milk are given in the C and D appendixes. If you suspect that food allergies are responsible for your child's allergic reaction, putting the youngster on an elimination diet may tell you what is causing the problem. However, it is well to note that the diet is extremely boring. Children (and adults, too) have a hard time adhering to it. They must stick to it religiously; that is the only way to make it work. Beyond that, with the enormous range of foodstuffs and their variability, the diet may fail to turn up any suspects. An elimination diet can help in diagnosis, but it is a drawn-out and crude process and there is always the chance that it may not pay off in the end.

You may have a hunch as to what foodstuff is causing your child's hypersensitivity reaction, either because you have fairly good circumstantial evidence linking fast-developing symptoms to a specific food or because you had your child follow an elimination diet. To be sure you do have the food responsible, your doctor may then want to do a *challenge test*.

In conducting a challenge test, the doctor will put samples of the suspected food and something innocuous that looks exactly like it — a placebo — in capsules. The child will take either placebo or suspected agent on a number of occasions and will then be observed closely to see if the reaction occurs. (Neither the child nor the doctor will know what is being administered; this "double blind" procedure is a routine precaution to rule out the possibility that subjective feelings of either patient or physician will affect the results.)

In summary, the diagnosis of food allergy or hypersensitivity — identifying the agent or agents that cause the symptoms — can be a difficult and often unsuccessful enterprise. A direct, clear, and unmistakable link between trigger and symptoms occurs perhaps in one case in five; for the remaining cases, an elimination diet followed by a

TABLE 4
Foods Causing Hypersensitive or Allergic Reactions in Children

FOOD	MOST COMMON REACTIONS
Milk	Diarrhea, abdominal pain, hives, skin rash, wheezing
Eggs	Abdominal pain, hives, wheezing
Cereals (wheat especially)	Hives
Nuts	Hives, wheezing
Legumes (peanuts, soybeans)	Hives, wheezing
Shellfish	Hives, wheezing
Tomatoes	Diarrhea, abdominal pain, skin rash
Berries	Hives, wheezing
Citrus fruits	Diarrhea, skin rash
Melons	Itchy palate or eyes

properly conducted challenge test is the surest way to an accurate diagnosis of the cause.

ALLERGY- AND INTOLERANCE-CAUSING AGENTS

Almost anything taken by mouth can cause a reaction in some susceptible person. This infinite potential for mischief makes it difficult to pin down the exact cause of an individual allergic or hypersensitive intolerance reaction. There are, however, a number of foods or materials found in foods that are well known for their ability to provoke reactions.

Foods that trigger allergic or hypersensitive reactions in significant numbers of children and the types of reactions they can cause are listed in Table 4. In addition, other substances found in food are often responsible for hypersensitive or allergic reactions. Table 5 names some of the more common agents, where they are encountered, and the symptoms they can produce.

In addition to what is ingested there are a few conditions the child may have that give the appearance of food allergy or intolerance, although they are really due to organic problems. These include enzyme deficiencies and GI tract diseases, notably gastric and duodenal ulcers, hiatal hernia, and inflammatory bowel disease. These causes are uncommon in youngsters but they do turn up occasionally.

In young children food intolerances or allergies are usually reflected in gastric complaints — colic, stomachache, constipation, diarrhea. Chapter 10 deals specifically with these symptoms, their incidence, causes, and treatment.

TABLE 5
Nonfood Substances and the Reactions They Cause

CAUSAL AGENT	FOUND IN	MOST COMMON REACTIONS
Mold	Cheeses; fermented meats; fermented beverages like beer, dried fruits, yogurt	Wheezing
Antibiotics (bacitracin, penicillin, tetracycline)	Meats, poultry, milk	Hives, skin rash, wheezing
Insect residue	Spices	Diarrhea, abdominal pain, hives
Herbicides, pesticides	Fruits, vegetables	Skin rash
Preservatives		
Sulfiting agents	Dried foods	Wheezing
Nitrates and nitroids	Preserved meats	Diarrhea, abdominal pain, wheezing
Sodium benzoate and benzoic acid	Ketchup, pickles	Diarrhea, abdominal pain, wheezing
Sodium proprionate	Stored meats and fish, many breads	Diarrhea, abdominal pain
BHA and BHT (butylated hydroxy-amerole and butylated hydroxytoluene)	Many dried foods such as dry cereals	Diarrhea, abdominal pain
Food coloring		
Tartrazine (yellow food dye #5)	Taco, potato, and other chips, dry cereals, some medication; ubiquitous	Wheezing
Flavor "enhancers" and sweeteners		
Monosodium glutamate (MSG)	Chinese and Japanese restaurants; packaged foods; other prepared foods	Diarrhea, abdominal pain, sweating, rapid heart rate
Texturing agents		**
Enzymes		**
Bleaches		**
Other chemicals		**
Bacteria and bacterial toxins		**

** The reactions are too few to categorize and not completely documented.

TREATMENT OF FOOD ALLERGY OR HYPERSENSITIVITY

To prevent the recurrence of symptoms brought on by a food allergy or intolerance, the obvious tactic is to avoid ingesting the substance responsible. Where a food or foods are implicated, this means not eating that food or, often, other foods that belong to the same family. (Food family groupings are given in Appendix B.)

Where chemicals or other additives or contaminants are concerned, avoiding the offending substance may be a bit more difficult. If the agents causing the reaction are additives, be especially attentive to content labels. The major sources of trouble are sulfiting agents that are used as preservatives and tartrazine, food dye #5. Appendixes D-4 and D-5 name some of the more common places where these additives are found.

A general procedure to follow in identifying foods or food additives or contaminants responsible for allergic or hypersensitive reactions is sketched in Figure 4 on page 75. Observing the steps and precautions spelled out there should enable you to keep your child from harm. Unless approved by your doctor, medications, especially over-the-counter drugs, should not be used to treat food intolerances.

TOO MUCH OF A GOOD THING

We have encountered food-linked complications in a significant number of allergic children. These children's life-styles seem to follow one of two behavioral patterns. *First,* some youngsters are kept needlessly sedentary, and their allergies are given as the reason. One result of enforced inactivity is overweight or in some instances obese youngsters. In allergic children this carries serious side effects. It undermines their developing the ability to resist or fight off some complaints like asthma, and it is associated with higher levels of vulnerability to allergy-linked complaints like chronic earache.

Second, there is a strong tendency for parents to think of a robust appetite as a sign of good health; accordingly, they ply their sick children with food treats and delicacies in the belief that food puts the child on the road to health and well-being. Food is not a medicine; a sound, sensible diet is necessary to good health, but merely consuming food will not cure anything. Forget folk sayings like "Feed a cold and starve a fever" or vice versa. It is upsetting to see the recent increase in the number of allergic children we treat who also show symptoms of bulimia, a psychological disorder marked by a morbidly increased appetite associated with recurrent vomiting. We have the sense that this pattern of eating behavior originates with the parents' excessive concern over the underlying allergic condition — usually asthma — and their unconscious attempt to treat it with excessive amounts of food.

TOO MUCH OF A GOOD THING

5.

Colds and Respiratory Infections

Colds are as much a part of childhood as Christmas or Sesame Street. Between the ages of two and four a child will typically experience 10 or more colds per year. It is misleading to use the word "cold," because cold symptoms (which can take many forms) can be produced by so many different kinds of viruses. The four major types of viruses known to produce upper respiratory diseases are respiratory syncytial virus, rhinovirus, parainfluenza, and influenza. Respiratory syncytial virus infections occur only in infants. There are nearly 100 different subtypes of rhinovirus, and numerous versions of parainfluenza and influenza that can infect individuals of any age.

Because of their numbers alone it is impossible to develop immunity to all viral respiratory infections; in fact, there is some recent evidence that immunity to certain viruses is only temporary and people can be reinfected time after time by the same virus.

These four major kinds of virus are of special interest to us because they have all been shown to make allergies, particularly asthma, worse. For nonallergic children, colds and other routine respiratory infections are benign, clearing up on their own in a few days' time. For the allergic youngster, however, some thought and attention needs to be given to the prevention of colds and respiratory infections.

PREVENTION OF COLDS AND RESPIRATORY INFECTIONS

There are many factors inherent in the body that are responsible for resistance to colds. In fact, one of the mysteries of medicine is why two people so very much alike in other respects, respond so differently to colds.

> Jack and Jerry live on the same block. They were both born in February of 1980 and are now eight years old. Jack hardly ever seems to get sick; Jerry, on the other hand, seems to catch every cold that shows up in the neighborhood and seems to keep it for longer than anyone else. Why?

Why is a good question, and one we cannot completely answer. Every reader knows that we have not as yet found ways to prevent or to treat the common cold. There are, however, specific factors that help to change how we develop infections. Inadequate nutrition, psychological stress, poor personal hygiene, lack of sleep or fatigue, recurrent diseases of the lung — all seem to be associated with more frequent respiratory infections.

THE IMPORTANCE OF GOOD NUTRITION

Americans have become a junk-food-ridden society. We eat junk breakfast cereals loaded with sugar and preservatives but lacking critical fiber and vitamins. We have fatty fast-food lunches that are about as well balanced nutritionally as the styrofoam containers they come in. We eat too many frozen and not enough fresh vegetables. We binge eat and drink. Is it any wonder that a significant percentage of our population has nutritionally associated lipid disorders in their blood (high cholesterol)? A number of studies have shown that many schoolchildren have marginal levels of zinc in their bodies, lack iron and other critical minerals and vitamins, and are anywhere from overweight to obese.

Having a well-balanced nutritional program is not necessarily going to prevent colds, but the person who is malnourished or not eating the "right stuff" is more likely to have common colds, and they will hang on longer than they do in people who eat properly.

PSYCHOLOGICAL STRESS

We do not know why individuals under physical or emotional stress are more likely to develop illnesses, but the connection is well known. A number of experimental studies in animals reveals that infections, and even cancer, develop more readily under stress. Stress in humans is also associated with increased incidence of injury or illness. We talk about stress and how to manage it in Chapter 22.

HYGIENE AND GENERAL HEALTH HABITS

Most people wrongly believe that colds are spread by one's being coughed or sneezed upon by a person already infected. Certainly being coughed or sneezed upon is not likely to foster good health, nor good relationships for that matter. However, the data now show that colds are *mainly* transmitted by hand contact; shaking hands, using communal towels, and so on. Since most colds are transmitted long before the person realizes he or she is infected, unceasing and unfailing preventive strategies must be followed in order to reduce the likelihood of contracting a cold. Here are some steps your children (and you) can take to cut the number and severity of colds.

1. Practice good health habits; get plenty of sleep, eat properly.
2. Keep in good physical shape; exercise regularly, watch the weight.
3. Avoid contact with people who are coughing or sneezing.
4. Do not get overheated; avoid drafts.
5. Drink plenty of fluids (at least one quart daily).
6. Ask the doctor about the advisability of flu or pneumovax vaccination (see Chapter 24).
7. Wash hands frequently during the day and always after using the bathroom and before meals; keep hands away from the nose, eyes, and mouth.
8. Do not share eating utensils or glassware; avoid public drinking fountains.
9. Have individual towels; do not use communal towels.
10. If you have a cough or cold, cover the mouth when sneezing or coughing.

RECURRENT OR CHRONIC LUNG DISEASES

There are other conditions that contribute to catching colds. One of these is underlying preexisting illness. Children with cystic fibrosis, a serious respiratory disease, have severe recurrent respiratory infections that often become life-threatening. Cystic fibrosis children produce too much thick mucus; the mucus clogs the airways and bouts of pneumonia often follow. Similarly, children with histories of recurrent pneumonias or those who have congenital defects that interfere with normal cleansing of the lung — those born with abnormal airways, for example — are also more likely to have their colds turn serious. Children with asthma seem to have more respiratory infections, which seem to get worse as time progresses.

Finally, smoking tobacco and using illicit drugs are not only dangerous practices but also make the user more vulnerable to respiratory infections. Parents who allow their children to smoke tobacco or dope are at best irresponsible and certainly negligent.

6.

Airborne Allergens

Airborne substances are the single most common cause of allergic reactions. In addition to provoking respiratory allergic symptoms in children — mainly seasonal or chronic hay fever or asthma — they may intensify complaints like eczema and they are often linked to other problems such as chronic earache, itchy, teary eyes, and gastrointestinal difficulties. The symptoms follow a period of sensitization and are uncommon in children before the age of four.

The most important airborne allergens are

- plant pollens
- molds
- dust
- animal dander
- smoke (especially tobacco smoke)
- pollutants (industrial or vehicular)
- other airborne particles (insect parts, soaps, detergents, and other household cleaning materials, chemicals)

PLANT POLLENS

Plants give off pollen as part of their reproductive cycle. The tiny pollen spores (thousands of them could comfortably occupy the head of a pin) invade the respiratory passages and, in the susceptible child, bring on the symptoms of hay fever.

You can broadly determine if plants are responsible for your child's distress by noting whether or not the symptoms are seasonal — and, if so, during what season they occur. If they turn up only during the early spring, chances are good that pollens are at fault — pollens from trees, in particular. If they appear late in spring or during the summer, grasses or weeds are more likely to be implicated. Appendix E gives the times when various kinds of pollens become airborne throughout the United States.

Not all plants give off allergy-producing pollens. Goldenrod, for example, once drew the blame for the hay fever that turns up in the late summer and early fall in the eastern and midwestern United States; ragweed, the real culprit, has the same blooming cycle but did not reap the blame initially because it does not flower as showily as goldenrod.

Chapter 12 tells how to control hay fever symptoms. When they are due to pollen, avoiding or minimizing contact with the offending substance is the most effective tactic, although difficult to carry out in practice. Air filtering devices are extremely helpful in cleaning out pollen; Appendix F describes types and features of various air purification devices and lists the best, most effective ones available.

MOLDS AND FUNGI

Breathing in spores from mold or fungi is another important cause of chronic hay fever or asthma in susceptible and sensitized youngsters. Molds occur both in- and out-of-doors, and a large number of them are capable of triggering symptoms. Establishing that they are at fault and identifying the one or ones responsible for symptoms is a difficult and imprecise business, because their sheer numbers make developing a comprehensive battery of tests next to impossible.

Fungi and molds thrive under warm, moist conditions. Consequently, they and the symptoms they cause are more likely to flourish during the warm, more humid seasons of the year. Major indoor and outdoor sources of mold and fungi are listed in Table 6.

Chapter 12 discusses control procedures for molds and fungi. Scrupulous cleanliness is important; in addition, if the symptoms are chronic and resist treatment, air purification devices and hypoallergenic decor in the bedroom of the affected person will likely prove helpful.

DUST

Dust, inside or out-of-doors, causes allergic reactions — usually perennial allergic rhinitis — in some youngsters. Parents cannot do much

TABLE 6
Sources of Airborne Molds or Fungi

INDOOR	*OUTDOOR*
Damp basements and crawl spaces	Leaf or plant surfaces (grasses, hay, and wheat-growing areas especially)
Bathrooms and showers	Decomposing (decaying) plant materials
Window frames	
Utility rooms	
House plants	
Rubber and foam pillows	
Vaporizing, humidifying, and air-conditioning equipment	

about outdoor dust except try to limit the child's exposure to it. House dust is a different and somewhat more manageable nuisance. While house dust contains a little bit of everything, its single most important component insofar as allergic youngsters are concerned is the dust mite. The dust mite primarily inhabits fabrics — carpeting, upholstery, cloth wall hangings, curtains and drapes, mattresses, blankets. It likes warm, humid conditions. It subsists on bits of skin shed by humans; inhaling the insects themselves or their waste matter triggers the hay fever-like symptoms.

Cleanliness — particularly of the bedroom — is the key to control of allergies triggered by house dust mites. In addition to the general control measures given in Chapter 12, here are some specific things you can do to get rid of dust — and dust mites.

1. Use plastic shades or blinds instead of curtains and drapes.
2. Remove rugs, any fabric wall hangings, overstuffed furniture. Replace with plain wood or plastic.
3. Keep clothes in a closet. Keep the closet door shut.
4. Clean every other day, using a damp cloth or mop to pick up dust. Do not sweep or vacuum. Pay special attention to dust-catchers like radios, TVs and other electronic gear, books, bureau drawers.
5. Beware of toys, especially plush or stuffed dolls. If there are any (current fashion seems to call for the child's bed to be buried under a mound of them), send them away on a *long* visit.
6. Use hypoallergenic bedclothes (mattress and pillow cover, sheet, blanket) *if necessary*; see Appendix J for suppliers.
7. Control temperature and humidity with a room air conditioner. (Keeping the relative humidity at less than 50% will kill the pests.)
8. Install an air cleaner *if necessary*; see Appendix F for recommendations.

ANIMAL DANDER

Animals are responsible for a good deal of misery in allergic children. By animals we mean not only cats and dogs — horses, rabbits, hamsters, mice, rats, and birds are also known to be responsible for the chronic hay fever symptoms shown by vulnerable people.

Nor is it just the animals themselves — their food and water dishes can harbor mold or fungi; they carry parasites that can be troublesome in their own right; bird droppings dried and dispersed are known to cause serious lung disorders; and even some pet food ingredients can trigger a reaction. What appears to do the most damage, however, is breathing in dried dead skin cells, whatever the species, and dried saliva (from cats cleaning themselves). The make of animal (small, large, shorthair, longhair) seems unimportant; it is not the hair but what's under it that mainly causes the problem.

The safest pet for an allergic child is a Pet Rock. (Even fish tanks sprout mold that can provoke sniffling or wheezing.) For allergic children, the most prudent course is to keep no pets at all, to avoid contact with other people's pets, and to take preventive measures when going into a situation where animals were or are present. Medications that can block reactions to animal dander and other animal-induced triggers and the strategies for using them are given in Chapter 12.

SMOKE

Smoke frequently causes asthmatic symptoms — wheezing and shortness of breath. Any type of smoke can be responsible, but the most common villains are tobacco smoke, smoke from wood-burning stoves or fireplaces, and candles. If your child is sensitive to smoke, the obvious course to follow is to see to it that he or she has as little contact with it as possible.

Cigarette smoke is the major source of trouble, and if the child is bothered by it, house and automobile should be declared smoke-free zones — easier said than done. (Even if children are not sensitive to cigarette smoke, they should be spared exposure to it; the damage to lungs from ambient tobacco smoke extends far beyond triggering wheezing.)

Quitting smoking where as powerfully addictive a drug as nicotine is involved is a severe test of fortitude and will. Yet millions of Americans, recognizing the mortal danger of the habit, have been able to do it. If you have not succeeded, now may be the time to expend the effort that will see you through; your Health Maintenance Organization and local American Lung Association office offer information about quitting smoking.

If wood smoke associated with home heating affects your allergic youngster, you can at least minimize the problem by making sure that the stove is tight and well vented to the outside. Clean, unobstructed stovepipes and an adequate draught ought to ensure that the house itself is largely smoke-free.

Candles or incense, since they are burned largely for ambience or decor, can be readily discarded. If the birthday cake has to have a candle, keep it to one. The symbolism will be preserved; more important, so will the health and well-being of the child.

POLLUTANTS

Industrial and vehicular emissions are responsible for respiratory problems, too. They are more likely to be a significant factor in urban, industrialized settings — most of the major cities in the United States have occasional to near-permanent periods of moderate to severe air pollution. Even Denver, once a haven for asthma sufferers, has a perennial smog problem. Strategies to follow in coping with air pollution are spelled out in Chapter 11.

OTHER AIRBORNE ALLERGENS

Robby, six, loves to go to the supermarket with his mom. She is understandably reluctant to have him along, partly because, in a supermarket, almost any six-year-old is a loose cannon, and partly because Robby always goes into a violent fit of sneezing and coughing when they pass down the aisle where the soaps and detergents are shelved.

The environment has been invaded by literally thousands of chemicals, many of which can become airborne and cause respiratory symptoms of one kind or another. Most airborne chemicals that cause problems emit pungent odors. Thus, it is more often an irritant effect than an allergy. Clearly we have much to learn about the role of chemicals in allergies. Until we do, parents of children troubled by chemicals will have to learn how to deal with the symptoms they produce through trial and error — possibly with some help from the doctor.

7.

Weather, Climate, and Exercise

In addition to the myriad of substances that can cause allergic reactions, many allergic children also have to contend with the fact that the mere accident of being or doing can provoke or worsen their symptoms. Extremes of heat or cold, the seasons of the year, and the level of activity of your child — all can and often do bear on allergic symptoms.

COLD

Exposure to cold in and of itself can trigger or worsen asthma or hives directly. Wearing wool, leather, fur, or down garments to keep warm can also start a child wheezing or itching with eczema or contact dermatitis.

Cold air is a major problem for asthmatics. Sometimes just the act of stepping outside on a cold day is enough to induce bronchospasm.

> Ben, 10, has had moderate asthma since he was 2. He lives in a small town near Buffalo, New York, which is justly renowned for its harsh winters. One extremely cold, snowy, and windy Sunday, he and his mom, dad, and younger brother are returning home from church. The car hits an icy patch and slides off the road into the ditch. His mother and brother are slightly shaken up. The father stays to minister to them and instructs Ben to run to a nearby house for help. As soon as he gets out into the frigid gale, Ben starts wheezing. His wheezing seems to get worse with each step he takes, and he barely manages to get to the house which is only 300 yards away

from the car. By this time his breathing is so bad that when his knock is answered, he is unable to say what the trouble is and, almost in shock, can only point outside and gasp "Help!" The householder immediately senses the trouble, has Ben come into the warm house, and telephones for help to go to the accident scene.

This wheezing problem can be controlled by adopting tactics that warm the air before it gets to the airways — filtering it through a scarf or ski mask, for example.

Hives can be caused by many physical, environmental factors — see Chapter 14 for the various causes. It is especially important to understand cold-induced urticaria (hives) because it is quite common and can become so severe that its victims have to bundle up literally all winter. Any lapse will result in children developing hives and enduring the maddening itching that accompanies them. Indeed, the symptoms can become more generalized and cause severe shortness of breath, even a shock reaction.

Tom has had cold-induced urticaria for three years. He is now 12 and enjoying summer camp — or at least he was until he jumped into the lake. The water felt cold as soon as he hit it and he knew that he shouldn't have done it. Within seconds his body started to swell and itch and he got *very, very* short of breath. That was the last thing he remembered. His camp counselor said he was lucky to be alive and only survived because it happened to be the day of the doctor's weekly visit to the camp. His prompt and effective action saved Tom's life.

Tom's near-fatal reaction is rare, but when a reaction like this does occur, sudden immersion in water is often responsible. To control cold-induced hives, see to it that your child dresses appropriately and avoids sudden exposure to cold air or water.

HEAT

Extreme heat can be particularly troublesome for children with eczema. These children are warned to keep from sweating and overheating — warnings that are difficult if not impossible to enforce. But the plain fact is that excessive heat dries the skin and causes it to crack and itch; it also induces sweating, which can make the skin irritable, especially where it comes into contact with clothing. Eczema flourishes under these conditions and should be managed along the lines sketched in Chapter 13.

HEAT AND COLD

Some children suffer chronically from a condition known as vasomotor rhinitis. While this is not an allergic complaint, youngsters with it have snuffly noses throughout the year, and the snuffles are made worse by breathing in air that shows any significant extreme. Going out into the cold will start the nasal faucet running; even sniffing a hot mug of soup can be troublesome. (Vasomotor rhinitis is discussed in Chapter 12.)

Oftentimes a humidifier is prescribed as a remedy for vasomotor rhinitis. This approach is usually ineffective and, as we point out in Chapter 20, can put the child at risk to mold allergies if the device is carelessly or improperly maintained. About the only thing a parent can do when confronting this problem is to teach the child to carry a good supply of tissues and to blot — not blow — the flow. (Blowing, which tends to force mucus into the sinus cavities, is associated with sinus infections.)

BAROMETRIC PRESSURE AND HUMIDITY

Changes in barometric pressure and humidity level, along with the temperature, affect asthmatics. Asthma is inversely related to all three of these features of climate, that is, the lower the humidity, temperature, or barometric pressure, the greater the likelihood of bronchospasm. As the nineteenth-century American essayist Charles Dudley Warner once observed, "Everybody talks about the weather but nobody does anything about it." There's not much you can do about the weather outdoors, but you can maintain a comfortable temperature and a good level of relative humidity — 60–70% — indoors. (Keeping to this standard should also reduce the risk of eczema, and energy costs as well.)

The susceptibility of asthmatics to low humidity and cold is one reason we recommend swimming. Exercise or activity under these conditions does not seem to precipitate wheezing.

THE SEASONS

As any hay fever sufferer knows, a year has two seasons — hay fever time, and the rest of the year. Depending on the plants responsible, hay fever can turn up at any time during the growing season. Since parents can't stop the plants from growing or children from playing outside, they are left to take the preventive and control measures that are spelled out in Chapter 12. The main thing is to be aware of when the problem is due to turn up and to prepare for it appropriately.

ACTIVITY AND EXERCISE

Exercise or activity in itself can induce asthma. It can also provoke hives and cause eczema to appear or worsen. With asthma, the type of exercise and the conditions under which it is done has an important bearing on events. Sustained exertion under dry or cold weather conditions will almost certainly bring on wheezing. Asthmatics should avoid jogging or distance running; swimming (as already noted), working with weights or weight apparatus, and other short-burst activities ordinarily carry no significant consequences.

Medicating appropriately will usually forestall exercise-induced asthma. Chapter 11 goes into the strategies to follow. However, it is important to note that there are two other aspects of exercise-induced asthma, something allergists and chest physicians are becoming increasingly aware of. The first of these is a delayed response where the bronchospasm does not occur until several hours after the exercise is over. The reason for this is unknown, but the existence of the phenomenon reminds us of the need for asthmatics to be judicious about exercise — to stick to what is appropriate for them and to be scrupulous about following preventive measures.

The second complication is that exercise can have a synergistic or additive impact on asthmatic children. Thus, if your child's chest is already tight from a cold or allergic asthma, exercise-induced bronchospasm can make matters worse, even to the point of making a trip to the emergency room necessary.

Finally, there is a rare disease known as exercise-induced anaphylaxis (EIA) that includes wheezing, hives, and shock. A small number of children are so bothered by exercise that anaphylaxis can follow exertion. Although the condition is extremely rare, its existence underscores the fact that what is simple fun to most can add up to tragedy for an unfortunate few.

8.

Skin Irritants

Skin irritation — dermatitis — is commonplace; almost all children show various kinds of skin rashes or outbreaks as they grow up. Their rashes may have any of a number of causes and may take any of a variety of forms. The most common ones are those arising from contact with one of the literally thousands of substances capable of causing the skin to erupt. A red rash, blisters, or hivelike wheals — all with or without itching — may be the result.

There are different classes of agents responsible for skin outbreaks in children. The age of the child has a good deal to do with which one is responsible and the form the symptoms take. The relationships between the age of the child and the nature, location, cause, and character of skin problems are described fully in Chapter 17. In most cases contact dermatitis is not an allergic reaction, even though there is a well-exercised tendency to label it as such.

Joel, a high school student and a computer whiz, helps out in the family business. He spends most of one weekend working with his father to set up a new accounts receivable and billing program. That Sunday evening he notices that his hands and face have become quite inflamed, red, tender, and itchy. He and his folks are mystified by this development until they review the weekend's activities and recall that Joel spent most of that time sorting through stacks of pressure-sensitized invoice copies. Joel is simply hypersensitive to one or another of the chemicals with which the forms are impregnated, although he and his folks like to say that he is "allergic" to them.

During earlier and simpler times dermatitis did not represent as much of a problem as it does today. While parents have always had diaper rash or poison oak to contend with, what makes the problem larger, more baffling, and more difficult to manage is the accelerating invasion of all parts of the environment by chemicals. These substances, whose aim is to make life easier, often have the effect of rendering it exactly the opposite. Hardly a day passes without a new — or "improved" — household product being thrown on the market. Cleaning agents, waxes, polishes, solvents, stain preventives, stain removers, and a bewildering variety of other household products keep turning up.

These manufactured substances are found everywhere — at home or school, in the workplace, in the automobile. They occur in fabrics, leathers, jewelry, and cosmetics; they are components of printer's ink, glue, toys; ironically, they are even found in some topical medications.

And, in addition to this constantly growing number of man-made irritants is the almost limitless number of naturally occurring ones.

> Carla, six, accompanies her mother to the library one fine morning in early spring. While her mother is inside, Carla amuses herself by climbing a low-branching olive tree in the library's backyard. Books found and checked out, Carla's mom collects Carla and sets off to run the rest of the morning's errands. They don't get completed, though. In about 30 minutes, Carla develops an itch followed by a case of hives involving much of her body and has to be rushed home. Her reaction to the heavy pollen and sap of the blooming tree clears rapidly, however. By evening she is able to resume her outdoor play.

The beneficial effects of the manufactured, fabricated products are trumpeted insistently — some of the miracles claimed for them may even be true — while their negative impact on the health and well-being of some users gets the silent treatment. To ask whether or not the product is capable of causing an itch or a rash in the user is a nuisance to the manufacturer. It probably can — almost anything will, given a susceptible individual — but looking for and then issuing a warning about any possible harmful side effects would run costs up and harm sales. To be perfectly honest, many manufacturers show little or no concern over whether their product represents a hazard to consumers.

Given this "let the buyer beware" attitude, what steps can you take to protect your youngsters from developing skin irritations? Here are some tactics you can follow that will at least reduce the risk or minimize the consequences of coming into contact with dermatitis-causing substances.

1. Be familiar with the forms the most common skin irritations take and their causes (see Chapter 17).

2. When a rash develops, be especially attentive to where it occurs on the body.
3. Review the child's activities carefully to try to pin down a cause for the problem.
4. Apply first-aid measures that will relieve the rash and the itching or pain that usually accompanies it.
5. Help the child to recognize and avoid whatever is causing the symptoms.
6. Be alert to the possibility of a secondary infection developing; if one does, consult your physician at once.
7. Help the child deal constructively with the problem in a supportive, stress-free atmosphere. Keep in mind that the youngster doesn't want the problem, didn't get it deliberately, is probably suffering acutely, and, since it is not contagious, can't give it to anyone else.
8. If the condition persists for more than a few days or shows signs of worsening, see your doctor.
9. Remember, most skin irritations are minor, short-lived, easily managed, and have no permanent adverse effects on either appearance or general health.

9.

Insect Stings or Bites

INCIDENCE

Allergic or hypersensitive reactions to insect stings or bites* are fairly common; just how common nobody knows. Individuals showing moderate to severe reactions or developing secondary infections to stings or bites are among the more frequently seen patients in the doctor's office or clinic.

USUAL AGE OF ONSET

Almost everyone, upon being stung or bitten by an insect, shows some sort of reaction, but its severity will vary greatly from person to person. Stings or bites causing more than slight, temporary discomfort (slight, temporary discomfort is by far the typical experience) can and do occur at any age. As a general rule, however, the intensity of the reaction is directly tied to age or to the number of prior exposures. Thus, individuals over 18, or who have had frequent encounters with the insect and have become sensitized to it, are the ones most likely to show trouble-

*Inhaling dust or debris that contains insect matter — wings, hair, body material, waste — can also cause reactions. See Chapters 6 and 12 for information about airborne allergens and how to deal with them.

some reactions. Infants or small children, while not unknown to have serious reactions, are the least likely to turn up with them.

SYMPTOMS

There are literally thousands of different insects, and many of them sting or bite humans. Table 7 names and lists the symptoms associated with the small number of insects responsible for most of the bite or sting problems encountered in the United States.

After your child is bitten or stung by an insect he or she will likely run to you complaining of symptoms in vague, general terms. Sometimes the child (and you) will be quite unaware that an insect is responsible for them. The location of the lesion and its appearance and characteristics (see Table 7) should help you to assign blame for the injury with reasonable accuracy and to take appropriate action.

HABITATS OF STINGING AND BITING INSECTS

Honeybees, wasps, hornets, and yellow jackets are found throughout the United States. The fire ant belongs to the same insect family as the bees, wasps, and so on, but is confined to the 13 southeastern and Gulf Coast states.

As for biting insects, mosquitos, biting flies, bedbugs, lice, fleas, scabies mites, and ticks are also found throughout the United States. Chiggers live in the Southeast and Southwest; wheel bugs occupy the area south of New York State, west and south to Texas; kissing bugs are prevalent in the South, Southwest, and along the Pacific Coast.

FIRST AID AND HOME TREATMENT OF INSECT STINGS AND BITES

Figures 2 and 3 trace first-aid and home-treatment measures to follow for insect stings and bites. You will see that there is some overlap in the charts — pain, swelling, and itching, whatever the cause, call for similar remedies. Moreover, when reactions can become general or life-threatening the need to seek emergency attention applies to both stings and bites.

We have given the best and most up-to-date ways of treating stings and bites. There are scores of other remedies, but little or no evidence that they are as sure and as safe as the ones we have mentioned.

TABLE 7 Stinging and Biting Insects and the Symptoms They Cause

STINGING INSECTS	STING SITE	SYMPTOMS		
		IMMEDIATE	1–20 MIN.	20+ MIN.
Honey bee,[1] wasp,[1] hornet,[1] and yellow jacket[1]	Exposed parts of body	Sharp, intense pain	Wheal at sting site, inflammation	Local swelling, itching, inflammation
Fire ant[1,2]	Exposed parts of body	Sharp, intense, burning pain	Blister or blisters at sting site, inflammation	Local swelling, itching, inflammation

BITING INSECTS	BITE SITE	SYMPTOMS		
		IMMEDIATE	1–20 MIN.	20+ MIN.
Mosquito	Exposed parts of body	Brief, barely noticeable prick	Wheal and inflammation at site	Small, itchy lesion
Fly	Exposed parts of body	Sharp pain	Wheal and inflammation at site	Small, itchy lesion
Wheel bug[1]	Hands and arms	Sharp, intense pain	Swelling, inflammation	Swelling, itching, inflammation
Kissing bug[1]	Face, hands, arms, legs	None	Itching at bite site	Swelling, intense itching, inflammation
Bedbug[1]	Face, hands, arms, legs	None	Itching at bite site	Swelling, intense itching, inflammation
Chigger	Legs and feet	Sharp pain	Wheal and itching at bite site	Small, itchy lesion
Flea	Feet and legs	Slight prick	Itching at bite site	Small, itchy lesion
Crab louse	Pubic area	None	None	Itchy lesion develops after infestation
Head louse	Scalp	None	None	Itchy lesion develops after infestation
Gnat	Exposed parts of body	Pain	Itch, swelling, and pain	Swelling, inflammation
Scabies mite	Much of body	None	None	Itchy lesion develops after infestation

[1]In extremely sensitive persons, may produce any or all of the following symptoms: hives and intense itching over much of the body, feelings of faintness, swelling of mucus tissue in throat, wheezing and difficulty in breathing. If any of these symptoms occurs, seek emergency help immediately!

[2]The fire ant is also capable of administering painful bites with its powerful jaws. The stings often form a circular pattern of small burnlike blisters around the bite site.

FIGURE 2
First Aid and Home Treatment for Insect Stings

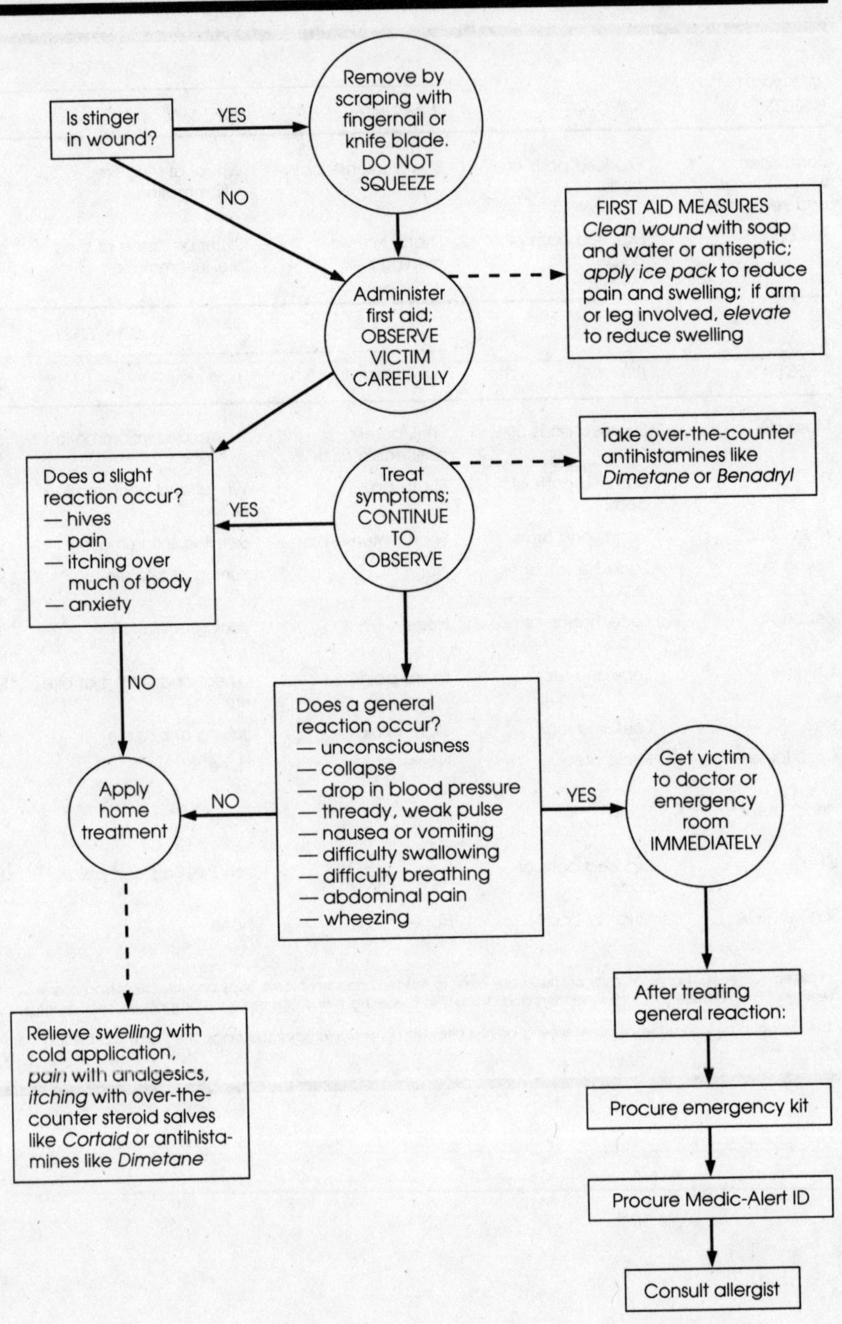

FIGURE 3
First Aid and Home Treatment for Insect Bites

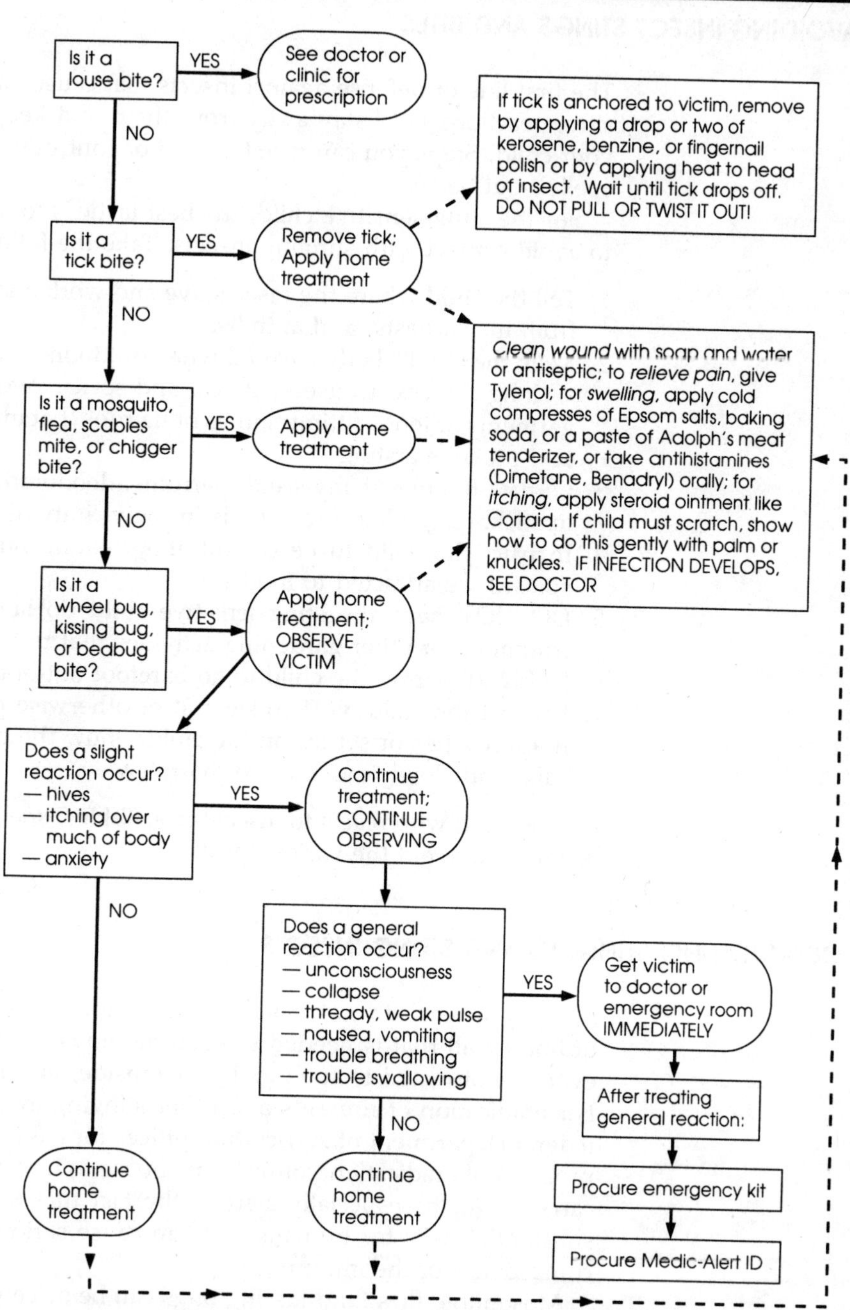

AVOIDING INSECT STINGS AND BITES

The first line of defense against insects that cause allergic or hypersensitive reactions is to stay away from them and keep them away from your child. Steps you can take to avoid or control these insect pests are spelled out below.

For the sting-sensitive child, the best tactic is to teach the youngster to avoid contact with stinging insects. Take the following precautions:

1. Tell the child where the insects live and work and how to stay away from hives, nests, and anthills.
2. Keep the child's body covered when outdoors during the bug season — long sleeves, trousers, shoes, and socks. Avoid brightly colored garments or loose-fitting clothes or hairdos that might trap the insects and provoke a sting.
3. Outlaw the use of any scent (perfume, deodorant, cologne, powder, lipstick, etc.) when the child is in the vicinity of stinging insects.
4. Instruct the child to be careful about eating out-of-doors as some species are attracted to foods.
5. DO NOT have the sting-sensitive child do lawn mowing, hedge trimming, or other gardening activities that put him or her at risk.
6. DO NOT permit the child to go barefoot out-of-doors.
7. Instruct the child NOT to swat at or otherwise provoke an insect if it approaches or settles on the child. Show the child how to remain calm and slowly move out of harm's way.

For the child who reacts to insect bites, Table 8 spells out steps that can be taken to avoid the various pests.

CONTROLLING STINGING AND BITING INSECTS

Stinging insects do not usually invade houses, and tight screens are ordinarily all that is needed to keep the house secure. Fire ants, however, are attracted to food and, once inside, are difficult to eliminate. For eradication of fire ants and other stinging insects, consult state or federal Department of Agriculture offices for advice. If you decide on a program of eradication yourself, or choose to hire a pest control firm to carry it out, be especially alert to the fact that many pesticides carry substantial risks for humans and can cause serious damage including compromise of the immune system.

Mosquitos, flies, and kissing bugs can be screened out effectively. If fleas, lice, bedbugs, or kissing bugs do get established indoors, scrupulously cleaning the places they inhabit is usually enough to get rid

TABLE 8
Avoiding Biting Insects

TACTIC	FLIES AND MOSQUITOS[1]	CHIGGERS	WHEEL BUGS	FLEAS	TICKS	MITES AND LICE
Use a repellent containing diethyl-toulamide[1]	X	X			X	
Keep body covered — wear slacks, long sleeves, shoes, hat; avoid loose clothes or hairdos that could trap the insect	X	X	X		X	
Do not use scents or perfumes, lotions, cologne, deodorants, etc.	X	X	X		X	
Insect-proof your pets				X	X	
Avoid contact with individuals infested with the pest						X

[1] Thiamine, vitamin B_1, available in health food stores and pharmacies, is thought to act as a mosquito repellent, but it can sometimes cause side effects — itching, hives, rash — and should be used with caution.

of them in time. The Department of Agriculture has free pamphlets available which give detailed instructions on how to be rid of these nuisances. Wheel bugs, ticks, and chiggers are outdoor pests. They are difficult to control, although their numbers can be reduced to some extent by keeping vegetation trimmed, eliminating trash, and storing wood neatly — and away from the living quarters. As with stinging insects, insecticides to get rid of biting insects should be used cautiously, as a last resort, and with careful observation of the warnings that pesticide manufacturers are required to make known to users of their products.

LONG-TERM TREATMENT

If your youngster reacts severely to insect stings or bites, take whatever precautions are necessary to prevent exposure. If the reaction is dangerous or life-threatening (rare but not unknown in children), here are some additional steps you should take.

1. Obtain, learn how to use, and have an ANA-Kit available and ready for use at all times. (Your doctor will have to prescribe this kit, which contains antihistamines and a syringe preloaded with epinephrine.)
2. Have the child wear Medic-Alert identification, which will signal and specify the existence of a possible problem to anyone called upon to administer emergency treatment. (Medic-Alert applications and information can be picked up in the doctor's office or clinic, by writing

the Medic-Alert Foundation, P.O. Box 1009, Turlock, CA 95381-1009, or by calling (209) 668-3333.)

3. A series of shots can desensitize your child to attacks by honeybees, wasps, hornets, yellow jackets, fire ants, or kissing bugs. The procedure — see Chapter 24 for details of how allergy shots work — almost always succeeds in reducing the severity of reactions to stings or bites dramatically. Talk to your physician or allergist about the possibility and appropriateness of desensitization for your child.

COMPLICATIONS

The two major complications associated with insect stings or bites are infections brought on by scratching and, in a few instances, anaphylactic or shock reactions brought on by the sting or bite itself. To control itching, follow the treatment directions given in Figures 2 and 3; if infection does develop, consult your physician promptly.

Anaphylaxis occurs in individuals who are extremely susceptible to certain antigens. It has been known since the time of the pharaohs that bee stings can cause serious or even fatal reactions in some individuals. This anaphylactic or shock reaction can also be caused by injections — allergy shots are the most common cause, but penicillin, novocaine, and other medications and a long list of foods are also capable of provoking this swift and dangerous response.

The anaphylactic reaction occurs rapidly — sometimes in a matter of seconds — and is marked by some or all of the following symptoms: massive outbreak of hives; swelling of mucus tissue, especially of the mouth and throat; wheezing or respiratory compromise; vascular collapse leading to a drop in blood pressure; faintness, or even loss of consciousness; nausea and vomiting; and feelings of anxiety, confusion, or dread.

This dangerous reaction requires immediate countermeasures. The standard treatment is to inject epinephrine, which reverses the drastic drop in blood pressure, and to administer antihistamines, which counteract the massive histamine release that is central to the problem.

If your child does go into shock when exposed to insect stings or other agents, you should have and know how to use an ANA-Kit, which you can buy with a prescription from your doctor. The kit should be kept available for immediate emergency use at all times and it should be fresh. It is prudent to carry an extra kit in your car. In addition, have your child carry or wear Medic-Alert identification to alert medical personnel to the existence of the problem, whatever its cause is, in the event of an emergency. The Medic-Alert Foundation's address is given in the preceding section.

A SPECIAL NOTE ABOUT SPIDERS

Many people fear or dread spiders and wrongly blame them for bites or stings actually delivered by other culprits. Only a couple of North American spiders — the black widow and brown recluse varieties — are dangerous. Their poisonous bites need to be treated *immediately* with antivenom serum, which is available in hospital emergency rooms and clinics. Note that children, because of their smaller body size and weight, are more likely to be endangered by the bites of these spiders.

PART THREE

THE COMMON ALLERGIC DISEASES, WHY CHILDREN DEVELOP THEM, AND THE STEPS YOU, THE PARENT, CAN TAKE TO DIAGNOSE, TREAT, CONTROL, AND AVOID THEIR SYMPTOMS

10.

Gastrointestinal Complaints (Colic, Constipation, Diarrhea, and Stomachache)

At some time in their lives most children are likely to turn up with gastrointestinal problems — colic, constipation, diarrhea, or stomachache. In Table 9 we have outlined these conditions, the usual age of onset, the symptoms, and their causes.

One especially common problem in infants and young children is recurrent colic. In small babies this condition can be severe enough to cause extreme stress in the parents.

> Tammy seemed like a normal baby until she was eight weeks old. Then, she started waking up virtually every night at one o'clock in the morning, irritable, restless, and crying. Nothing her parents did seemed to make her comfortable. They discussed it with their pediatrician, who recommended they eliminate milk from her diet. For 10 days immediately thereafter, Tammy's colic improved; then it started again exactly the same way it was before. Finally, at five months of age, the colic disappeared, and Tammy's parents were at least able to get a decent night's sleep. Those three months were the worst ones they had ever experienced.

Milk allergy was strongly suspected in Tammy's case, but her experience did not indicate that milk was unequivocally involved. Allergy to eggs is likewise common in children. Egg allergy, like milk allergy, can produce everything from eczema to wheezing to hives to abdominal pain.

Establishing the causes of these various gastrointestinal or stomach disorders in children is difficult because they are manifold and obscure.

TABLE 9
Common Gastrointestinal Complaints in Children

CONDITION	*USUAL AGE OF ONSET*	*SYMPTOMS*	*CAUSES*
Colic	Infancy, birth–6 months	Abrupt severe crying, clenched fists, drawing of knees to chest, flushing, tense and distended abdomen	Not fully known; often associated with sensitivity to milk
Constipation	Infants, children, adults	Infrequent or incomplete bowel movements, irritability, lethargy, loss of appetite	Various; most commonly associated with dietary deficiencies, obstructions
Diarrhea and vomiting (immediate hypersensitivity reactions)	Infants, children, adults	Diarrhea, vomiting, nausea, abdominal pain and distension	In infants, associated with food intolerances, especially to milk, egg whites, nuts, seafoods, some fruits; also caused by GI infections, parasites, maturational delays, enzyme insufficiencies, and many stomach flus
Chronic stomachache	Children 5–10	Intermittent, recurring pain which can be cramping, dull, or sharp and localized; usually located near the umbilicus	Not fully known; attributed to food allergy, constipation, abdominal, migraine, irritable colon, psychological

For that reason there is a well-established tendency to blame them on allergies — in particular, food allergies.

CAUSES OF FOOD ALLERGIES AND INTOLERANCES IN CHILDREN

Virtually any food or drink can trigger an adverse reaction in a susceptible child. The symptoms may constitute a true allergic reaction and take any of the varied forms that characterize allergies — wheezing and shortness of breath, hives, angioedema (see Chapter 14), eczema, hay fever — as well as the gastrointestinal complaints listed in Table 9, and sometimes, the generalized, systemic life-threatening response of anaphylaxis. Male children, by a two-to-one margin, appear to be more prone to these allergic reactions; susceptibility to them probably owes much to heredity.

There is a wide variety of foods, food colors, food preservatives, and preexisting conditions in the individual that can also produce symptoms that closely mimic allergic reactions; in fact, these account for most negative reactions to food testing (see Chapter 4). This mimicry makes specific diagnosis extremely difficult.

The diagnosis of a true allergy, as we noted in Chapter 1, requires the presence of the antibody IgE. This IgE binds onto special white cells known as basophils or mast cells, and under appropriate circumstances (such as eating the food one is sensitive or allergic to), these white cells release histamine and the other chemicals responsible for the allergic reaction. However, there are ways that allergens can cause white cells to release histamine and chemicals directly *without* IgE involvement. A large number of foods and drugs are capable of doing this. The best example of this is seen in a sensitivity to berries — strawberries, in particular — in children. Sensitive children, if they eat berries, develop GI problems, itching, hives, or even a full blown anaphylactic reaction. This sensitivity to berries often disappears as the child gets older. This may be due to changes in the way that people digest their food as they grow older.

> Sherry experienced her first bout of hives when she was five, shortly after eating strawberries. She and her family quickly learned that berries make her very sick and produce itchy skin bumps. When she was 25 she decided to try a taste of fresh strawberry pie. To her surprise and delight, she was no longer sensitive.

Actually, the substances mainly responsible for these peculiar non-IgE reactions are food dyes and preservatives. The best studied of these is tartrazine, the yellow food dye found in tacos, potato chips, some capsules of medicine, some toothpaste, and more products than most people could find imaginable. Persons who are hypersensitive to tartrazine may also be sensitive to aspirin (salicylates), too. (See Chapter 4 and Appendixes D-2 and D-4.) This is an important issue, which needs further study.

FOODS ASSOCIATED WITH GASTROINTESTINAL SYMPTOMS IN CHILDREN

The foods that appear on a list of the leading causes of food hypersensitivity (and GI troubles) in children depend on the expert doing the listing. While there is common agreement on the importance of cow's milk, eggs, shellfish, nuts, and wheat as provokers of reactions, the unanimity stops with them. Legumes (peanuts and soybeans) are frequently mentioned, as are fish and mollusks. However, the authorities disagree on the role of tomatoes, chocolate, and citrus fruits, which are popularly identified as *allergens,* even though strict laboratory experiments have failed to support this charge. (Chocolate can make your child sick, but it is not borne out that the sickness is allergy-caused.)

The most important nonfood triggers of GI problems in children are:

- Enzyme deficiencies in the child
- Antibiotic contaminants (bacitracin, penicillin, tetracycline) found in meats, poultry, or milk
- Insect residues found in spices
- Chemical food additives, including monosodium glutamate (MSG), metabisulfite, and tartrazine
- Bacteria and bacterial toxins

A NOTE ON MILK AND ENZYME DEFICIENCIES IN CHILDREN

Cow's milk is by far the most common reason for food sensitivity problems. This is not surprising considering the enormous quantity of milk consumed by children, helped along by the earlier trend (now beginning to reverse) toward the use of bottled milk and milk-based formulas in preference to breast-feeding. Thus, a much larger proportion of infants in the past two generations were bottle-fed than had been at any previous time in world history. Some call this the largest uncontrolled experiment in the history of civilization.

Cow's milk, whether whole, low fat, or dry, contains many proteins. It also contains lactose, which is its principal sugar. A substantial percentage of blacks and Asians are born with a reduced amount of the enzyme lactase in their intestines. (This lack also shows up in young children of any ethnic origin.) Because they do not have an adequate amount of lactase to handle it, the milk sugar often passes undigested out of their stomachs. Transfer to the bowel may therefore be rapid and lead to considerable bloating, stomach pain, diarrhea, and excessive gas. This is an intolerance, not an allergy to milk. Lactase deficiency may also turn up in other people of any ethnic background who stop drinking milk for a few months.

IDENTIFYING FOOD INTOLERANCE

A strategy to follow in identifying the food (or the myriad of additives, contaminants, or other conditions) responsible for your child's hypersensitive reaction is sketched in Figure 4. The chart outlines what is essentially a conservative and minimally risky series of steps to follow. *The key to successful attainment of the information you need is careful observance of an elimination diet.* A general elimination diet, together with the steps you will need to follow to see it through to a successful conclusion is presented in Appendix A. Following the procedures outlined in Figure 4 and sticking faithfully to the elimination diet, if it is called for, should point to whatever is causing your child's food intolerance. The

FIGURE 4
Steps in the Identification of Food Hypersensitivity or Allergy

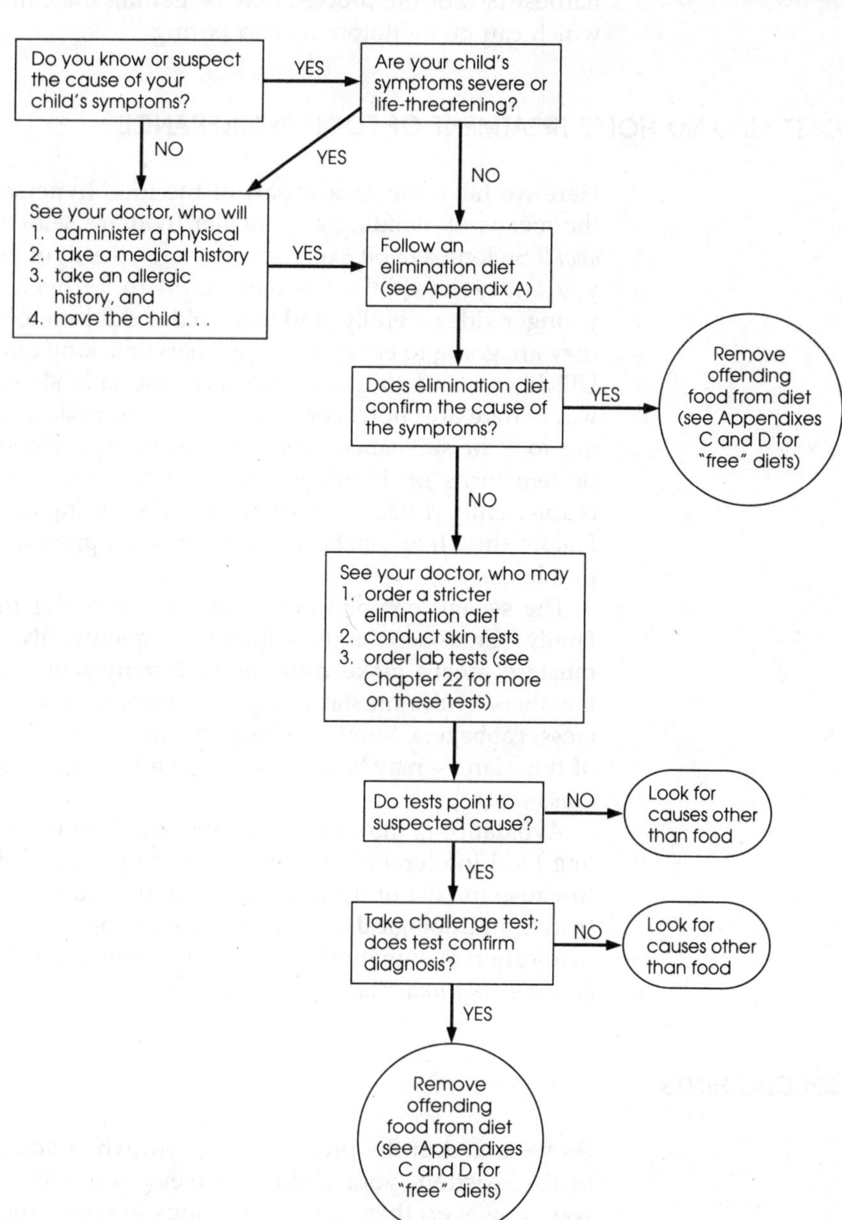

hardest part of the process may be getting the child to stay on the diet, which can be monotonous and boring.

FIRST AID AND HOME TREATMENT OF FOOD INTOLERANCE

Here we have the easiest part of the food hypersensitivity scenario — the means of avoiding a particular food are self-evident. Avoid means *avoid!* So long as you exercise a certain amount of vigilance and caution, you and your child's troubles ought to be over. Monitor the diet of younger kids carefully, and teach older children to find out exactly what they are going to eat by reading labels or asking questions. DON'T SLIP UP! If you and they exercise care, the kids should be out of harm's way. There are, however, two possible complications: First, the offending food or substance may occur in unexpected places. (Milk or milk protein turns up in everything from bologna to zabaglione; tartrazine is apparently ritually cast into nearly everything processed or prepared.) Follow the "free" diets in the C and D appendixes to sidestep these problems.

The second complication is that the offender may come from a big family. Cross-sensitivity happens frequently in food intolerances. If mustard greens make your child's tummy ache, for instance, all of the members of the mustard family — turnip, radish, horseradish, watercress, cabbage, Chinese cabbage, broccoli, and the many other members of this clan — may also do so. Appendix B gives families of foods that cross-react.

Avoidance is the safest and most effective tactic to follow in controlling food intolerance symptoms. If complete avoidance is not possible (because the list of irritants is long and diffuse) and if the sensitivity is truly immunological or allergic, then suppressing symptoms through medication is sometimes a workable alternative. *This control step should be taken only under medical supervision.*

SPECIAL HINTS

As we noted in the preceding section, when you do isolate the source of the reaction, your child's problems are over — almost. Along the way, however, there are a few things to know and to be careful about.

A special problem occurs in young children. As we pointed out above, infants and young children often absorb small quantities of food that remain undigested. As children grow older, however, their gastrointestinal tracts mature, food comes to be digested completely, and absorption of small quantities of undigested food no longer occurs.

With this maturation of the intestine and proper food digestion, the symptoms of food allergy generally disappear. However, if these children go on to develop pollen sensitivity (hay fever), their food allergies may return.

DO NOT permit skin tests or oral challenge tests if the child's food intolerance is severe or life-threatening. Skin tests (scratch or prick) for food hypersensitivity are crude, cover only a small fraction of the possibilities, are potentially dangerous, and are useful mainly in their ability to identify *lack* of sensitivity to a substance. A course of skin tests will likely eliminate some suspects, turn up a few false leads (false positive reactions), and, only perhaps, the real culprit. Challenge tests are the key to definitive identification of specific causes of food hypersensitivity. (See Chapter 4 for more on challenge tests.)

[illegible] simpler forms of allergy, generally disappear. However, [illegible] other [illegible] taken [illegible] that [illegible] changes may occur.

[illegible] of MCS patients [illegible] original challenge [illegible]

11.

Asthma (Wheezing and Shortness of Breath)

There are few, if any, ailments that terrify children and families more than wheezing and asthma.* Asthma accounts for more absences from school than any other chronic illness, and it is a leading cause of visits to doctors' offices. It is a serious disease — the death rate among hospitalized asthmatic children is under 1%, but rises to 2–4% in adults.

More than two thirds of asthmatics have a family member — brother, sister, or parent — who has or has had asthma, but the hereditary basis for the complaint is complex and not completely understood. Some children from families riddled with the complaint never show the disease; others from seemingly clear backgrounds inexplicably turn up with it.

INCIDENCE

Asthma (which originally meant "shortness of breath") is among the most common of ailments — up to 5% of Americans, 10 million people, suffer from it.

In childhood it is one third more common and more severe in males, but after puberty the sex distribution is about even. It is more often

*For a detailed discussion of asthma, its symptoms, causes, and treatment, see M. E. Gershwin and E. L. Klingelhofer, *Asthma: Stop Suffering, Start Living,* Addison-Wesley Publishing Co., Reading, Mass., 1986.

found in urban, industrialized settings, in colder climates, and among the urban disadvantaged, especially blacks.

USUAL AGE OF ONSET

Asthma may turn up at any age, although the first episode is likely to occur between the second and fifth years. In a few children, wheezing and shortness of breath are evident right from birth.

SYMPTOMS

Asthma is a collection of respiratory symptoms, the most prominent of which are shortness of breath, wheezing, coughing, and increased production of mucus. The shortness of breath (which can be sudden in onset) and the wheezing are produced by "twitchiness" of the respiratory airways.

As air is inhaled through either the nose or the mouth it flows through a series of airways. These airways — tubes, really — begin in the throat and descend all the way down to the base of the lungs. At the level of the throat and upper chest they are fairly large. The uppermost and largest is called the trachea. About one third of the way down into the chest, the trachea branches into two somewhat smaller airways known as main stem bronchi. Each of these main stem bronchi supplies air to one of the lungs.

As the bronchi extend deeper and deeper into the chest the air tubes proliferate and become smaller and smaller. The result is a complex maze of small tubes — airways — that resemble the root structure of a tree. Surrounding these airways is a layer of smooth muscle. This muscle maintains the size and shape of the airways. In asthmatics the muscle is "spastic" or "twitchy" — likely to go into a spasm when stimulated by any of a number of factors. When the smooth muscle sheath does go into spasm it chokes or constricts the airways, thus making less room for the air to move in and out of the lung. It is this restriction of airflow that produces the high-pitched wheezing and the struggle to breathe that are characteristic of asthma.

In addition to the layer of spastic muscle tissue around the airways, mucus-producing cells called goblet cells are important contributors to asthma. Everybody, whether normal or asthmatic, has these mucus-producing cells. Mucus is important because it carries the enzymes and chemicals that help the lungs to fight infection. In asthmatics, however, there is an increase in the number of mucus cells, with the number increasing with the severity of the asthma. These cells produce an excess of mucus, which clogs airways and obstructs the flow of air. This is especially true in the small airways at the bottom of the lungs.

CAUSES

Asthma has many different causes or triggers, both allergic and non-allergic. In children the most prominent ones are respiratory infections, airborne allergens, food additives, vigorous exercise, and exposure to cold, dry air. Asthma symptoms are also associated with cystic fibrosis (CF) and gastroesophageal reflux (GER), rare but grave conditions in infants and children.

WHEN TO SEE THE DOCTOR

Regardless of its severity, the very first wheezing episode should signal you to call your doctor even if the episode is mild and transient. At that appointment the doctor will take a medical history and carry out a physical examination, order a chest X ray, and, if necessary, give allergy skin tests.

A medical history and a complete physical examination are vital to the management of asthma. The physical should include measures of height, weight, blood pressure, and pulse and assessment of any other possible asthma-contributing factors. The chest should be very carefully listened to by the doctor to determine if there might be an anatomic basis for obstruction. A tumor or a foreign body in the airway causes a decrease in airflow and a wheeze. (Asthma is a symmetric disease affecting both sides of the chest; an obstruction is likely to affect only one side — perhaps only a section of one lung on one side. Careful listening can pick up this difference.)

At this early stage your child should have a chest X ray. It is usually not necessary to repeat chest X rays thereafter, but an initial picture will help identify any potential anatomic problems and will be useful for later reference. Following the physical examination, the physician and you must decide whether allergy skin tests are needed.

SKIN TESTING

Skin tests entail making a series of minor scratches or pricks on the skin and introducing different allergen extracts into these wounds; the substances to which one is allergic will quickly develop a raised, white patch with a surrounding redness of the skin.

Allergy skin tests that help to determine what is causing the wheezing and shortness of breath are among the most abused of all procedures in medicine. Many physicians, believing they are more accurate than they really are, carry out wholesale testing with allergic antigens. These antigens are often very crude; sometimes the test procedures irritate the skin and produce false positive results, that is, a reaction due not to an antibody or allergy but rather to a simple irritation that has nothing to do with allergy.

There are several factors that determine whether an asthmatic child should have skin testing. *Children under age four should be skin tested only under exceptional conditions*. If allergy skin tests are to be performed, which ones are administered should be determined by where you live and how the disease manifests itself. Allergy skin tests can be divided into several categories. The most common tests are those using pollens; the serums used are made from extracts of trees, weeds, and grasses. The child should be skin tested with pollens found in the locale — a Californian should not be tested with Midwestern weeds. Then, there are the mold antigens. Molds are found almost everywhere and many asthmatics are allergic to them. Third, there are the environmental agents that test reactions to things found in the home, especially house dust and animal danders. Finally, there are extracts that purport to detect sensitivity to certain foods. These last tests should be used rarely; they are very crude and unlikely to yield clinically important information. If food allergy is suspected, then the physician should carry out a special challenge test of the sort described in Chapter 6.

Occasionally, a bronchial challenge is carried out, usually in a hospital setting. If your youngster's symptoms are confusing or contradictory, he or she may be asked to inhale a vapor containing an allergen (often a pollen); sometimes the vapor will contain a chemical called methacholine. The reason for this test is to find out what causes the wheezing and to determine if the child really has asthma. Over 90% of asthmatics will show asthmatic symptoms when methacholine is inhaled; generally fewer than 10% of those who do not have asthma will have a positive reaction. If the results of the test are positive you can be fairly sure that your child does in fact have asthma, even though you and the doctor may still not know what is causing it.

TREATMENT OF ASTHMA

Effective treatment of asthma entails five rather complicated steps. Not all are applicable to everyone. The steps are

1. Identification of causal agents
2. Avoidance of causal agents

3. Control of appearance of symptoms through medication and other strategies
4. Treatment of symptoms
5. Prevention and/or reduction of symptoms through allergy shots

Identify the Causal Agent or Agents

Many factors can precipitate an asthma attack. The most important ones are

- Colds or upper respiratory infections
- Exposure to allergens
- Food additives
- Vigorous exercise
- Emotional responses, including hyperventilation
- Certain drugs, especially aspirin
- Air pollutants, including tobacco smoke, ozone, and sulfur dioxide

Some brief comments may help you in your search for the causal agent — or agents — responsible for your child's asthma.

Colds or upper respiratory infections are the most common forerunners of asthmatic attacks in children. The cold symptoms — sneezing, sniffling, coughing, stuffy nose, sore throat, possibly a slight fever — usually appear before asthma takes hold. Then the congestion will get worse, the chest will feel constricted, and shortness of breath, deeper coughing, and wheezing will show up. These asthmatic symptoms may persist well after the main infection is largely gone.

Allergies to pollens, house dust, animal dander, foods, and molds turn up in half of all asthmatic children, but they are not necessarily the major cause of their asthmatic reactions. Often, however, they are, if the child has a high level of IgE antibodies.

It is *food additives*, seldom foods, that cause asthma. Foods draw much unwarranted suspicion as causes of asthma. The idea that your child's asthma can be provoked by some mysterious, insidious allergy to foods is largely unfounded. Food additives though, can and do, particularly *tartrazine*, which is found in food dye color #5 (FD&C#5), a yellow dye used in potato chips, tacos, and other yellow candy and processed foods. Common foods containing tartrazine are listed in Appendix D-4.

Exercise is frequently implicated in bronchospasm. Interestingly, the form of exercise has much to do with it. Swimming is relatively harmless and unlikely to provoke airway collapse in asthmatics, while running or jogging often will. Whether or not exercise will cause your child to wheeze also depends on the temperature and humidity of the air breathed — the more moist and the warmer the air, the less the likelihood of wheezing. We encourage all children with asthma to become regular swimmers.

Emotional responses — anger and fear in particular — have long been blamed for causing asthma. While an emotional state like the anger or resentment that accompanies or follows conflict between parent and child does not induce asthma, it can cause rapid, shallow breathing or hyperventilation. This hyperventilation in children with twitchy airways brings on bronchospasm and wheezing. There are probably other ways in which emotional reactions induce bronchospasm — recent evidence hints at a relationship between personality traits and asthma. However, the underlying ways in which traits produce symptoms — if in fact they do — are still unknown.

Many drugs and particularly those classified as nonsteroidal anti-inflammatory drugs (aspirin and its relatives) can induce violent asthmatic reactions. If your child has asthma, steer clear of aspirin and all other nonsteroidal drugs.

Air pollution, especially from sulfur dioxide, ozone, and the particulate pollutants resulting from the combustion of fossil fuels, cause twitchy airways to get worse. In addition to atmospheric pollutants, tobacco smoke — first- or secondhand — is an important triggering agent for asthma and should be studiously avoided.

Avoid Asthma's Causal Agents

Once you identify the agents responsible for your child's asthma, the next step is to design effective ways of avoiding contact with them. Avoiding exposure to *colds and respiratory infections* is fairly difficult. (Chapter 5 spells out the steps you and your child can take to cut the risk of colds.) If vigorous *exercise* pushes your child into an asthmatic attack, he or she has three options; exercise anyway and suffer the consequences, substitute another activity, or take medication beforehand. For the first two alternatives nothing more needs to be said. If your child wants to do demanding sports or activities that provoke asthmatic reactions, Jim's experience may be instructive.

> Jim has had asthma all of his 15 years. He is particularly troubled by wheezing during physical exercise in school and is unable to keep up with the other boys on account of it. His doctor says that he has exercise-induced asthma and recommends that he take theophylline. Unfortunately, Jim cannot tolerate theophylline, which gives him an upset stomach and nausea, and he would much rather avoid exercise than take the medication. Jim's parents consulted another physician who recommended that he use an Alupent inhaler prior to exercise. Although school rules forbid students to carry hand-held nebulizers in their pockets, they are available in the school

nurse's office, so Jim goes there immediately before his gym class. Since he started doing this he has improved greatly in stamina, and, to his immense satisfaction, his athletic skills have picked up, too.

Asthma is a rich source of *emotional reactions*:

- Asthmatics and their parents experience frustration, fear, panic, and guilt over the attacks.
- Children having moderate to severe attacks spend a lot of time wondering if they are going to die this time.
- Parents understandably become oversolicitous and overprotective of their asthmatic children, keeping them from participating in and enjoying ordinary activities, from developing normally, and, in doing this, forging an undesirably close dependency that may be difficult to break in later life.
- Parents and nonasthmatic brothers and sisters quite often resent the attention, the care, and the expenditures that the asthmatic requires.
- Asthmatics may use their condition to have their way in the family or elsewhere.

If you establish that asthma in your child has an *emotional base* — if attacks have more than a coincidental relationship to other events that cause conflict, stress, anger, or frustration — teaching the child how to breathe when having an emotional reaction will help. The youngster should, at times of stress or tension, be taught to

1. Sit down in a quiet place. Turning the chair so that the child has nothing but the wall to look at is useful.
2. Take slow, deliberate, deep breaths, inhaling through the mouth and exhaling *slowly* through the nose.
3. Continue this for a short period of time — usually no more than five minutes should be enough to restore the youngster's ordinary breathing rhythm and reverse the bronchospasms.

To avoid some of the major difficulties growing out of emotional responses, keep communication lines open. Discuss problems frankly and directly as they come up. Do not let them fester. Do not treat your asthmatic children as invalids. If you do they may start believing you.

Any time your child sees a doctor or gets a prescription for *drugs*, remind the physician without fail that the youngster is asthmatic. By following three simple rules you can help your child avoid drug-induced asthma.

1. Monitor the child's reactions carefully after the use of *any* drug.
2. NEVER self-administer aspirin or any other nonsteroidal anti-inflammatory drugs or medications.
3. NEVER administer any drug without first letting your doctor know

about it and consulting him or the *Physician's Desk Reference* (available in public libraries and doctors' offices) for possible side effects — especially asthmatic ones.

The most common and serious of the *air pollutants* is tobacco smoke. ASTHMATIC CHILDREN SHOULD NOT SMOKE TOBACCO, THEY SHOULD AVOID THE TOBACCO SMOKE OF OTHERS, AND MEMBERS OF THEIR HOUSEHOLD SHOULD NOT SMOKE.

High concentrations of ozone and sulfur dioxide — air pollution — are the result of a conspiracy of climatic conditions and automobile emissions, which cause asthmatics considerable distress. Here is what to do if you and your child find yourselves in a smog-filled city.

Most cities with significant smog problems forecast air quality, and the index will appear in the morning newspaper. If the "smog" index is "high" or "alert," then it will be especially dangerous for your asthmatic child, because the pollutant indexes apply to normal people; people with respiratory disease start showing symptoms when the index is "moderate." When that happens, or is about to happen, keep your child indoors. Keep the windows closed. Have the youngster curl up with a good book or in front of the television set. Do not let the child play out-of-doors until the smog clears. If the youngster must go out then have him or her wear a disposable mask. Effective paper masks, much like those worn by surgeons or carpenters, are available at your drugstore. The mask will not affect the level of sulfur dioxide or other gas but will filter out some particulate matter. While outside in these conditions asthmatic children should not exercise or otherwise exert themselves. They should walk at a moderate pace and avoid other obvious triggering factors in the environment like automobile emissions and tobacco smoke.

Controlling or Treating Symptoms

Very often asthmatic symptoms — wheezing, shortness of breath, coughing — can be kept from developing or, if they appear, controlled by a combination of measures. These control measures include clearing the mucus, improving the airways through breathing exercises, and using medicine intelligently. The sections that follow tell you how you can put these measures into practice.

CLEARANCE OF MUCUS. During an asthma attack the goblet cells that line the airways drastically increase their production of mucus. When this sticky, tenacious material lodges in the airways it makes breathing even more difficult for your asthmatic child. Sometimes it gets so bad that asthmatics literally drown in their own phlegm.

There is nothing you can do to affect the production of mucus. There are, however, some simple and effective steps you can take to keep it thin and easy to move.

To keep mucus from getting dangerously thick and clingy, your child must drink *at least* two full glasses of water four times per day. Warm water is best for this purpose — stay away from juices, sodas, milk, and other beverages that carry the possibility of allergic complications and do not get absorbed by the body any faster. Spicy foods have also been found to loosen mucus. Adding 10 to 20 drops of Tabasco sauce to the water would be an appropriate dose for adolescent asthmatics. Getting the mucus *out* is a bit more difficult. However, it can be done readily enough provided you devote time to it and help your child in the process. What you will be doing, in fact, is getting the phlegm *down* and out, because you will have the child take a series of positions where the chest and torso will be higher than the head, and the mucus, aided by your gentle tapping, will be dislodged and ooze out of the airways. To do this you will need a stiff, wedge-shaped bolster a couple of feet square and at least four to six inches higher at one end.

Have the child lie on the bolster, belt line at the high end, head on the floor at the low end, back down, then left side down, then right side down, then front down (see Illustration 1).

In each position tap the uppermost part of the child's chest gently with your fingers. This will loosen the clinging mucus and speed its outward flow. A hand-held vibrator will also work (see Illustration 2).

For best results have the child stay in each position from three to five minutes. You will want to do the mucus clearing twice a day. Sleep will also be improved if you schedule one session just before the child goes to bed.

BREATHING EXERCISES. You can greatly reduce the severity of asthmatic attacks if you teach your child to breathe properly. There are three different kinds of exercises that will improve your child's breathing. The first kind teaches how to involve the diaphragm in the process of breathing — something that most people don't do.

1. Have the child locate the diaphragm (which is a large, powerful muscle) by putting the hands on the stomach between navel and rib cage (see Illustration 3a).
2. Keeping hands on the diaphragm, have the child take a deep breath. If the diaphragm is being used the hands will be pushed forward. Then exhale; the hands should now move inward (see Illustration 3b).

ILLUSTRATION 1

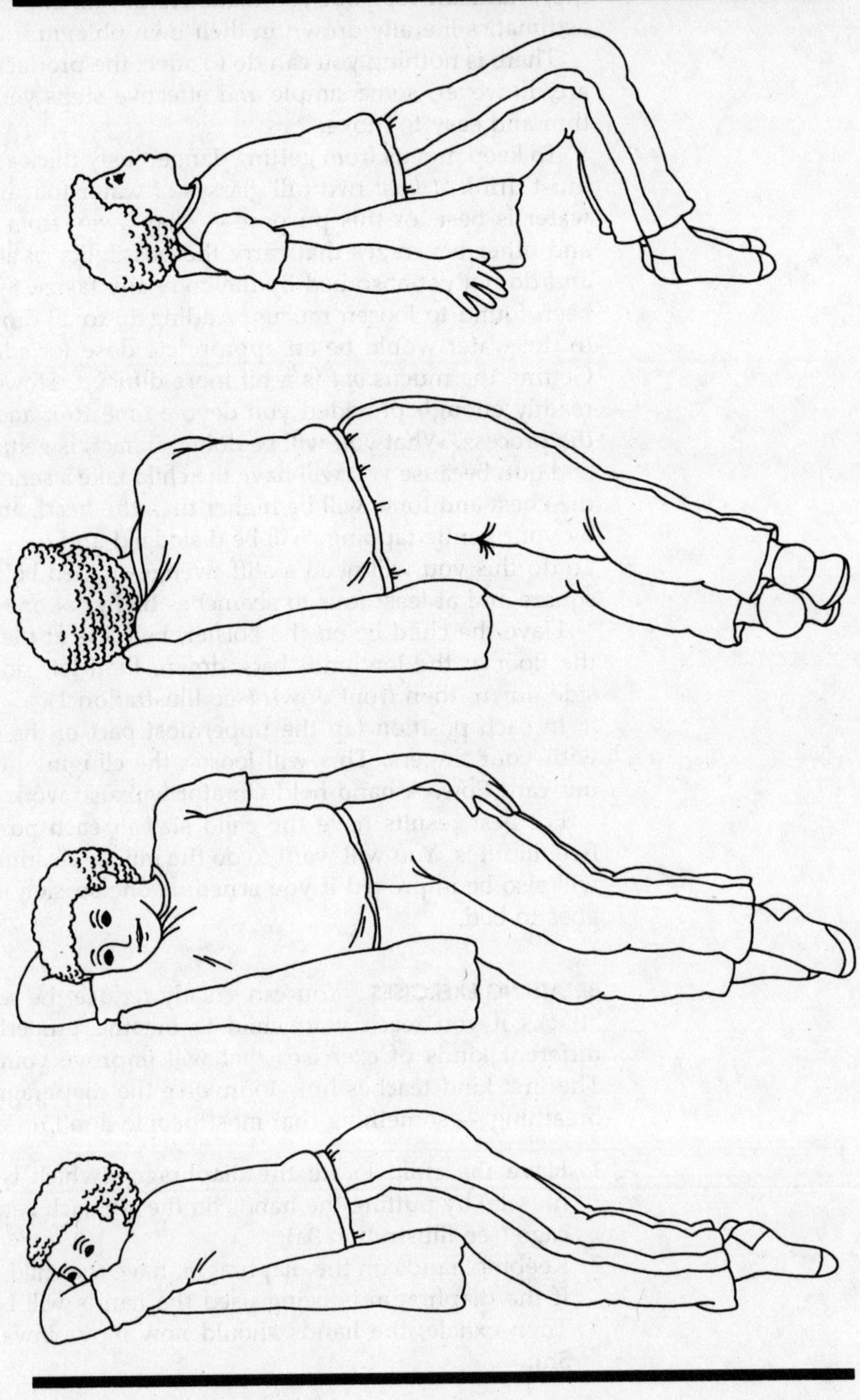

ILLUSTRATION 2

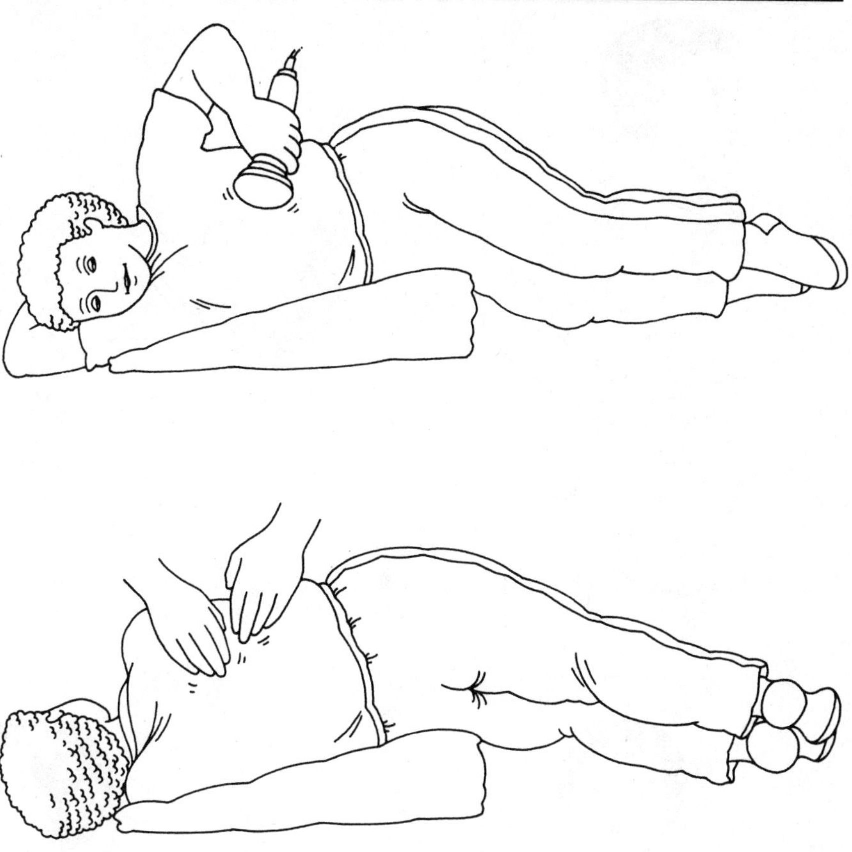

3. Once you get the child to the point where he or she can move the diaphragm, have the child practice diaphragmatic breathing four times a day for three or four minutes each time. Keep the hands on the diaphragm always; do the breathing exercise standing for one minute, sitting for one minute, and reclining on the back for one minute (see Illustration 3).
4. When, after a week or so, diaphragmatic breathing gets to be automatic, add this exercise. With the child lying on the back, place a weight — three to five pounds of books is about right — on the diaphragm. Have the child breathe in deeply, using the diaphragm, and then exhale slowly. Repeat this exercise 10 times twice daily. This will strengthen the diaphragm (see Illustration 4).

ILLUSTRATION 3

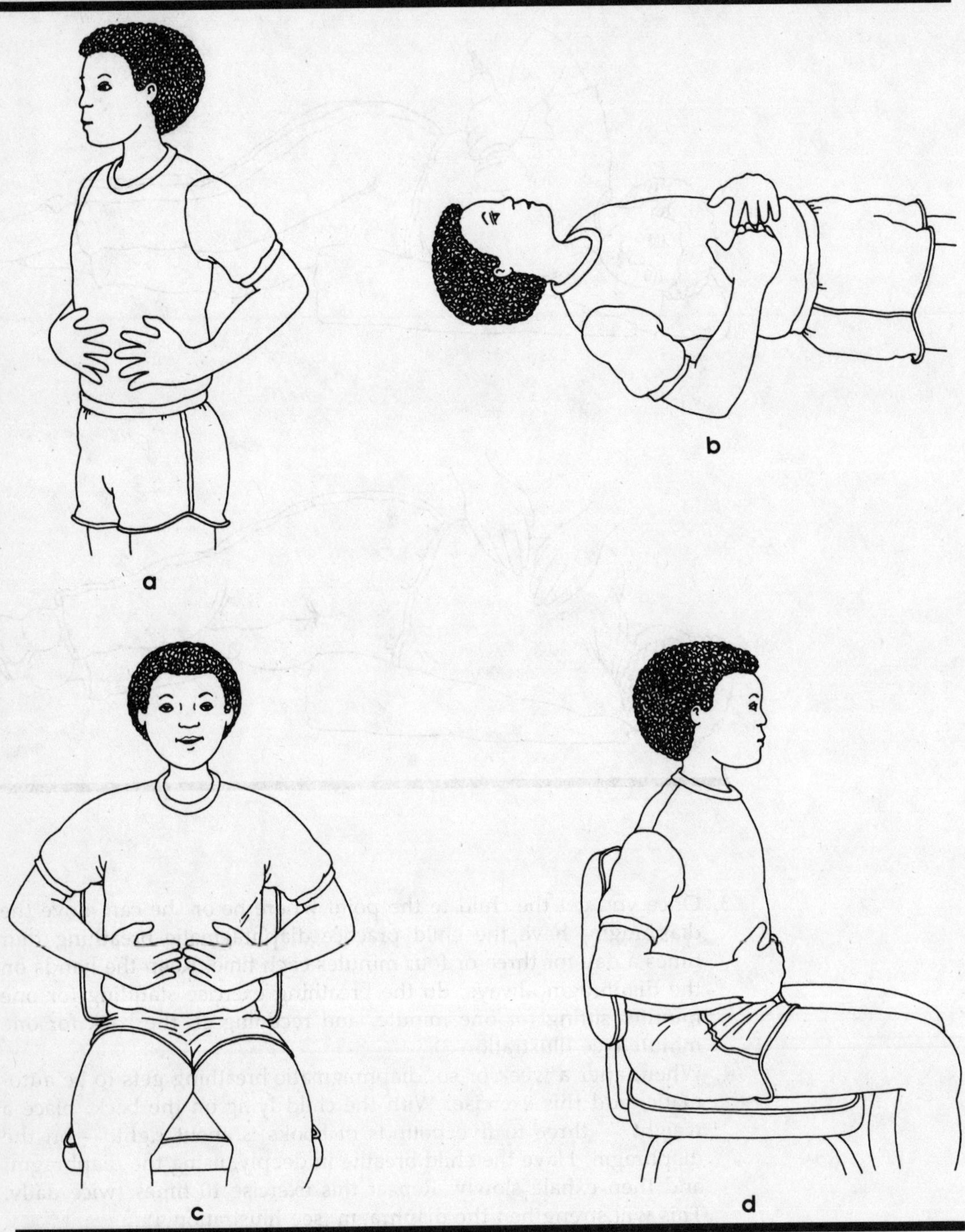

ILLUSTRATION 4

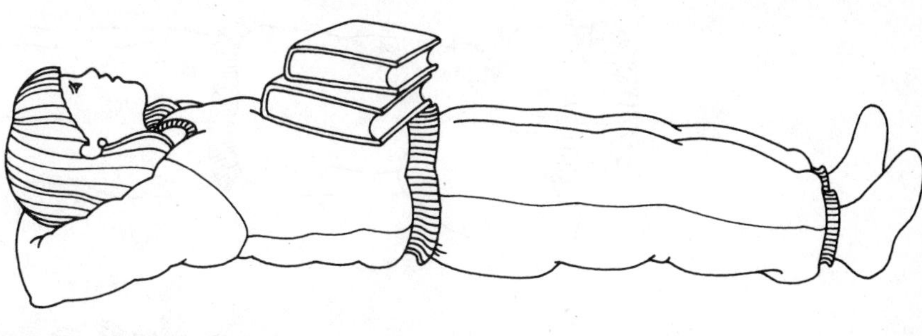

The second kind of breathing exercise helps expand the child's rib cage and get unused lung cells into action.

1. Have the child lock fingers behind the neck and press the elbows back while inhaling. Hold the breath a few seconds, then exhale while bringing the elbows together in front. (This exercise can be done sitting, standing, or lying down.) Repeat 10 times, twice a day (see Illustration 5).
2. Have the child sit upright. Raise the arms high while inhaling, then slowly bend forward and exhale slowly. The hands should touch the floor. Repeat 10 times twice a day (see Illustration 6).
3. Sit the child upright. Put one hand flat on the stomach and extend the other arm out horizontally and away from the body while inhaling deeply. Exhale slowly while bringing the hand of the extended arm to the opposite shoulder. Repeat, alternating positions of hands, 10 times twice daily (see Illustration 7).

As you know the bronchial tubes have walls of smooth muscle and it is this muscle that contracts and causes wheezing and shortness of breath. Your child's bronchial walls can be strengthened and made more resistant to spasm through the following exercise.

> Have the child clench the fingers of one hand so as to make a closed cylinder (the kind of arrangement you make when the hands are cold and you blow on them to warm them). See that the cylinder is as tight as possible. Have the child blow into it, remove it from mouth, inhale, blow again with increasing force. Do this for a minute or two three times daily (see Illustration 8).

These breathing exercises, if done faithfully, will increase your child's lung capacity, muscle tone, and resistance to asthmatic bronchospasm.

ILLUSTRATION 5

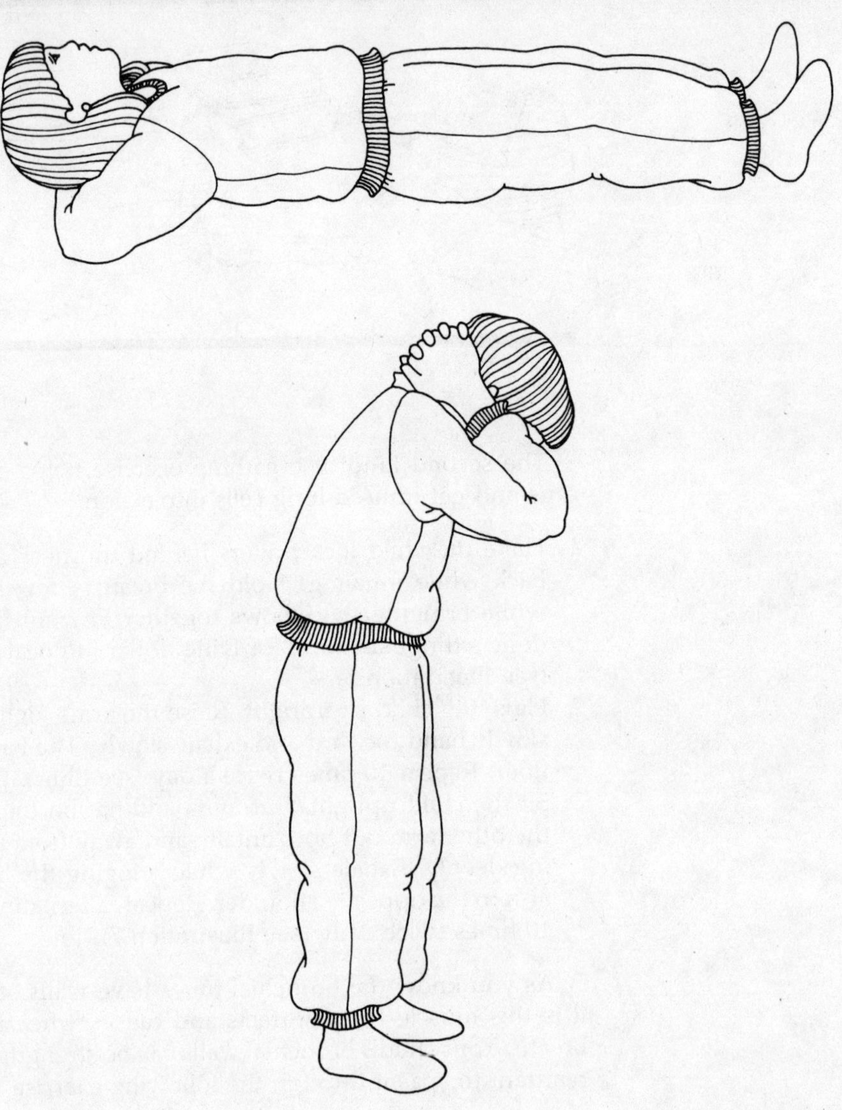

MEDICATION. There are several medications available that keep asthma symptoms from appearing or that relieve them when they are present. These medications are beta agonists, theophyllines, cromolyn, and corticosteroids (cortisone). Except for a few over-the-counter beta agonists,

ILLUSTRATION 6

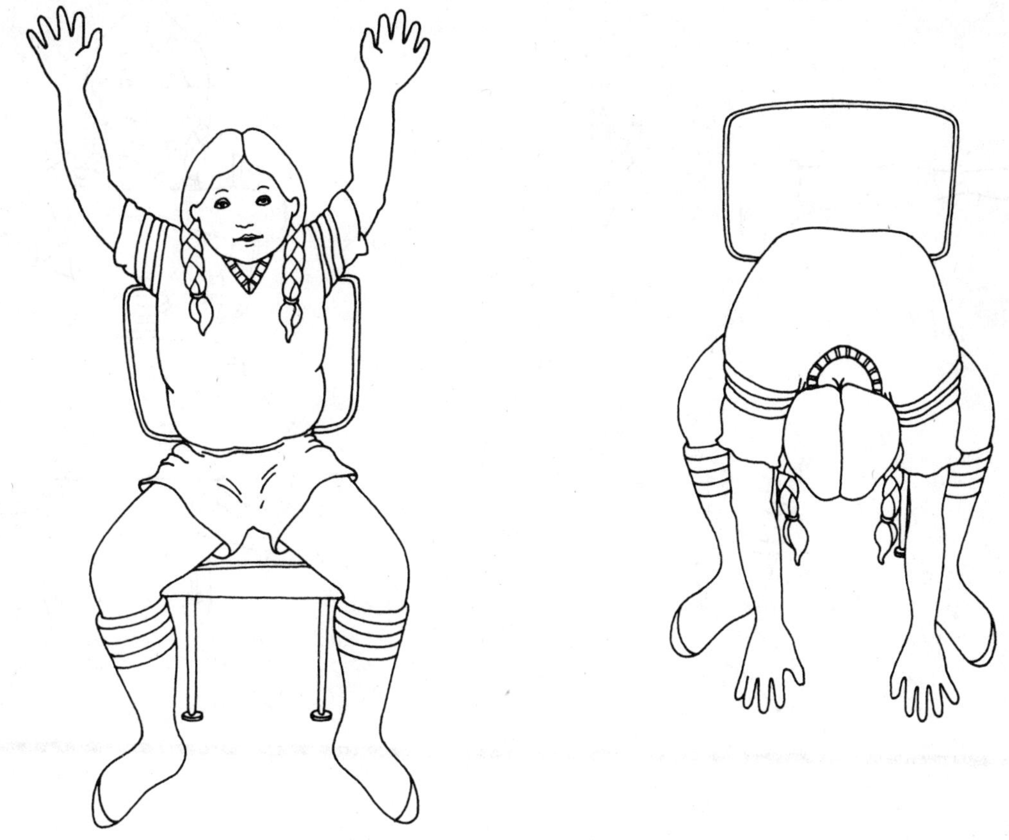

these are all prescription drugs and must be ordered by your doctor. They are appropriate for use if your child is moderately to severely asthmatic. The paragraphs below and Table 10 tell how the drugs act, what forms they take, the ages for which they are appropriate, and their advantages and disadvantages.

Beta agonists are the major class of medications for asthma. These drugs can be taken orally, but are most commonly and effectively administered by operating a metered, hand-held, aerosol canister. They provide rapid relief of asthmatic wheezing and shortness of breath. Activating the canister releases a puff of drug-saturated aerosol, which is carried directly to the twitchy smooth muscle in the airways. This

ILLUSTRATION 7

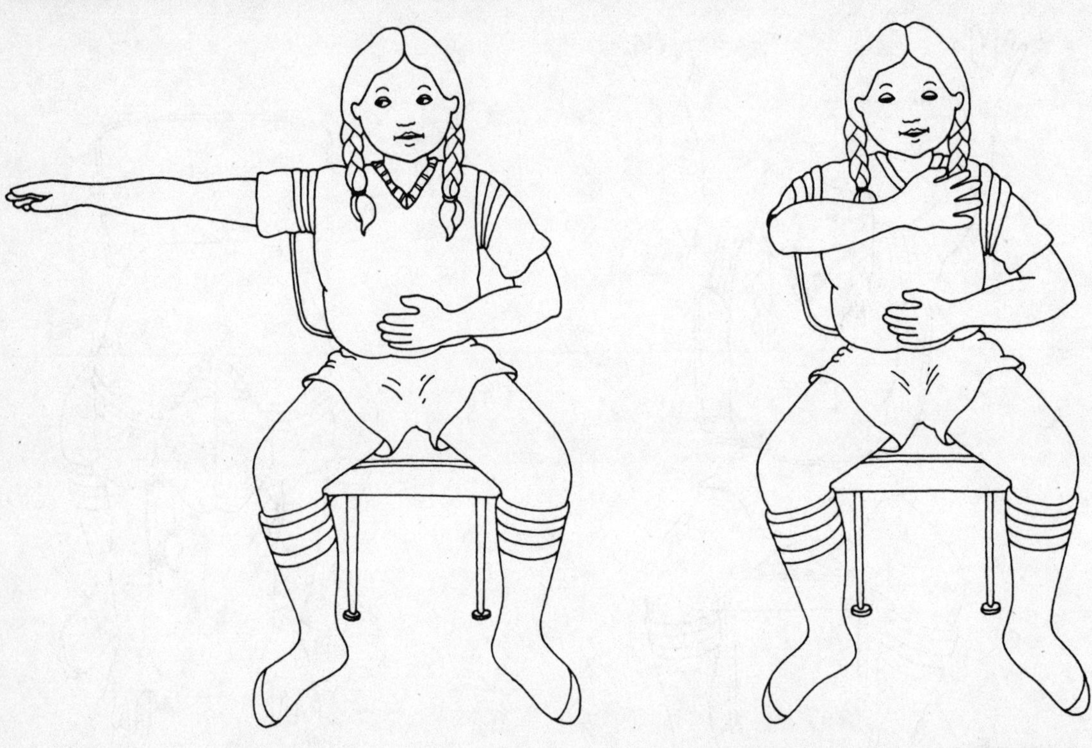

direct action quells the symptoms much more rapidly than the theophyllines do. Since they work almost instantaneously they are extremely satisfying to use.

Over-the-counter aerosols are available. Primatene Mist and Bronkaid, the two most heavily advertised ones, are effective for the treatment of occasional, very mild symptoms. They sometimes help children with mild asthma, but they are not as effective as new prescription drugs and are *more toxic*.

Beta agonists are the first line of treatment for asthma because they have fewer side effects, they are more convenient, and they act more rapidly. For more severe asthmatics and for very young children, we use solutions of beta agonists given by nebulization (see below) rather than the aerosol canister.

The effectiveness of aerosols depends very much on knowing how to use them. DO NOT OVERUSE AEROSOLS (1–2 inhalations every 4

ILLUSTRATION 8

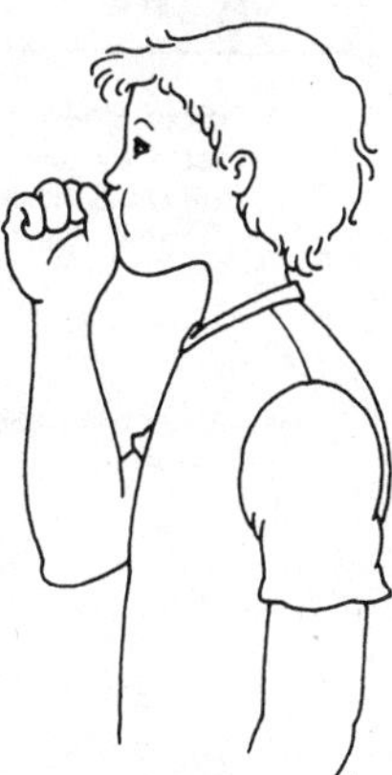

hours, and not more than 12 puffs per day, is enough). Teach your child the following steps in the effective use of a metered aerosol:

1. Shake inhaler.
2. Begin inhalation and, at the same time, place aerosol just in front of the mouth at a distance of one to two inches and release a properly aimed puff of aerosol (aerosol should go straight to the large airways; it should not impact at the back of the throat).
3. Inhale at a moderate rate with open mouth.
4. Hold breath for five seconds.
5. Exhale.

To direct the spray efficiently, "spacers" are often useful. A cheap, effective spacing device is the cardboard cylinder found within a roll of toilet paper. With seals between the mouth and the metered aerosol, it works quite well. A one-liter plastic container made into a simple cylinder has also been shown to be an effective delivery system. At least three commercial spacers are available — the Aerochamber (by Monaghan, Inc.), the Inspir-Ease (by Key Pharmaceutical), and the Inspir Chamber (by Schering Pharmaceutical). These devices cost between $12 and $16 and last for several months. The Inspir-Ease is the best.

These spacers simply hold the aerosol in suspension for several seconds. The child who is unable to inhale the aerosol successfully thus has more than one inspiration to get the medication to the lungs.

Theophyllines are related to caffeine and work by relaxing bronchial smooth muscle, thus opening up the airways and making breathing easier. The amount of theophylline to take depends on body size and has to be determined carefully. Even then there are sometimes signifi-

TABLE 10
Asthma Medications for Children

MEDICATION	*EXAMPLES*	*ADVANTAGES*	*DISADVANTAGES*
Theophyl-lines	Respid, Slo-Bid, Theodur, Theodur-Sprinkle	Effective drugs for mild and moderate asthma	Slow to act; strong stimulant affecting activity level and behavior; can cause sleep disorders; stomach upset; increase in urine output; sometimes toxic, especially when upper respiratory infections are present
Beta agonists	Alupent, Ventolin Max-Aire	Work quickly; convenient to carry; can be called into use as soon as needed; strongly recommended	Difficult to take effectively (see text); can, but seldom do, cause heartbeat irregularities, chest pain, muscle tremors, nausea, vomiting, dizziness, weakness, sweating
	Brethaire	Works quickly	Tolerance can develop; not recommended
	Bitoterol	Longer duration of action — to 6–8 hours	Takes 30 min. to work; *not* recommended
Cromolyn (Intal)	Powder	Very effective for allergy and exercise-induced asthma; few side effects	Can cause coughing and aggravate breathing difficulties
	Inhaler	Easier to use than powder	Sometimes not as effective as powder
	Nebulized solution	Dramatically improves delivery in young children	Requires a nebulizer
Steroids	Prednisone	Very good for severe asthma	Carries major and dangerous side effects; a treatment of last resort
	Beclomethasone, Azmacort	Act on lungs only; side effects minimal when taken properly	Not effective for acutely ill children; allergy to vehicle may develop; can trigger coughing and wheezing in some children
	Aero-Bid	None	Disagreeable taste
Anti-cholinergic	Atrovent	Low toxicity; may reduce cough	Not a first-line drug for asthma; best for chronic bronchitis in adults; most effective when given in combination with beta agonists

cant differences in reactions between like-sized individuals, so physicians, when prescribing theophylline, are likely to order a blood test, which measures how much theophylline is in the blood several days after starting to take it.

When taken regularly (and with careful initial monitoring of the blood to detect potentially dangerous side effects), theophylline keeps wheezing from developing and permits asthmatics to lead a much more comfortable and normal life.

Theophyllines come in four forms: (1) a liquid, (2) a chewable tablet,

(3) a pill, and (4) a capsule containing time-release beads. The liquid form, such as Slophylline, is very disagreeable to taste. The problem is found in all the theophylline elixirs and suspensions. They are definitely *not* recommended. The chewable tablets are only rarely better tasting than the liquid versions and are also *not* recommended. The tablets, such as Theodur and Respid, are preferable for older children.

The capsules, when swallowed, are just as good as the tablets. However, some capsules, such as Slo-Bid, can be opened and the beads spread over applesauce or yogurt, making it very easy for young children to swallow. There is even a special preparation of theophylline, called Theodur-Sprinkle, that is made just for this purpose. When using theophylline in young children, we recommend the bead or sprinkle, although your doctor must still check the child's blood to verify the levels of drug. Checking blood levels of theophylline is important for all patients. This is particularly valuable for young children as often the beads or sprinkles do not get absorbed.

Cromolyn sodium, a chemical originally isolated from an Egyptian weed, comes in three forms: (1) a powder which is inhaled, (2) a metered aerosol, and (3) a liquid for nebulization.

In taking the powder, a dose of the chemical is held in a capsule which is inserted in a "spinhaler." The spinhaler consists of a chamber, a cup containing a sharp pin, and a propellor fan. The pin pierces the capsule when it is placed in the cup. The asthmatic, by taking a deep breath, spins the propellor. The whirling propellor disperses the powder into the air that is being inhaled.

The metered dose of cromolyn (Intal) is administered in the same way as the beta agonists. The liquid for nebulization is given as noted below.

Cromolyn should be given a fair and serious trial by the young child! It is often not totally effective when given alone to control moderate to severe asthma. Thus, it works best when given with other drugs such as beta agonists. These comments aside, Intal is an excellent agent and has almost no toxicity.

Steroids, drugs in the cortisone family, are taken by children only when affected with very severe asthma — especially those who are hospitalized. Beclomethasone, a special topical steroid preparation, is available in an aerosol much like beta agonists so that, when properly taken, it acts only on the lungs. Unless it is used more frequently than recommended it does not produce the side effects of cortisone and can be quite effective in improving breathing. It does not deliver the amount of cortisone needed by severe (but unhospitalized) asthmatics, but, as a supplement to the other drugs named above, beclomethasone, which can be quite helpful, has its place.

Beclomethasone is usually prescribed as either Vanceril or Beclovent;

they are identical. Another topical steroid, Aero-Bid, is unpleasant to take because it has a bad taste and often induces nausea; it is therefore not recommended. Finally, a new topical steroid, Azmacort, is far superior to Vanceril or Beclovent because it comes with a spacer that greatly helps delivery. We have had such excellent responses with it that we sometimes call it "Amazing Cort."

NEBULIZERS. For very young children and for children who have very severe asthma, more effective and immediate treatment is often needed. About 10 years ago it was realized that a simple air compressor, when used to blow air through a solution of medicine, would create a fine aerosol of medicine — a nebula — which could be rapidly inhaled into the lung. The development of home nebulization equipment has been one of the most important advances in the management of asthma. The two most popular nebulizers are the DeVilbiss Pulmo-Aid and the Dura-Neb made by Dura Pharmaceuticals. Both of these units, available through medical supply houses, are excellent, although we strongly prefer the Dura-Neb because it operates from standard electrical outlets, the cigarette lighter in your car, or rechargeable batteries. These units cost from $175 to $350 and, when prescribed by your doctor, are paid for by most insurance companies. Patients who cannot afford them can often get them for free from local respiratory societies or rent them at a nominal cost.

> Chrissy, now 12, has had asthma nearly all of her life. For the first several years she had to have shots of adrenaline up to 30 times a year to control her symptoms. At age six, her doctor prescribed a Pulmo-Aid. Since that time, Chrissy has not required a single injection. She takes her Alupent as well as her Intal by nebulization and now plays softball, as well as the flute in the school band.

If your child is moderately to severely asthmatic, you *should* discuss the possibility and appropriateness of a nebulizer with your physician.

SPECIAL HINTS OR WARNINGS

It will help parents to note and remember the following points:

1. The belief that asthma is psychologically caused is a myth. If your child has asthma it is because of genes; nothing is the matter with his or her emotional life, although there may be, in time, if you act as if you believed the old misconception that asthma springs from psychological roots.
2. The most difficult aspect of asthma for parents is the acute concern,

sometimes verging on dread, they experience when they see their child fighting for breath in the grip of a moderate attack.

Note Carefully:

- The breathlessness usually seems more severe than it is. Don't panic.
- DO NOT advise the child to breathe deeply. This can actually make the symptoms worse. Let the child find his or her own respiratory rhythm.
- DO NOT encourage the child to cough. This can force mucus into the airways, further compromising the breathing.
- DO NOT administer any drugs other than the ones prescribed by your physician. In particular, NEVER give an asthmatic child sedatives, tranquilizers, or aspirin in *any* form (helping a child go to sleep can be extremely dangerous).
- Administer all medications exactly as prescribed in the amount and according to the schedule your doctor orders. (If you are not clear about what to do, clarify your responsibilities completely before leaving the doctor's office; do not undermedicate or overmedicate.)
- If the youngster's condition gets to the point where you can't help and seems to be worsening, don't hesitate to call the doctor or go to the emergency room. Wheezing is a serious sign and must be treated.
- Resist the temptation to seek treatment from chiropractors, herbalists, naturopaths, homeopaths, organic or psychic healers, or other unconventional "healers." They have nothing to offer that will effectively relieve the smooth muscle spasms that trigger asthma.

3. Be wary about putting your child through a course of allergy shots for the prevention of asthma. In no case should a young child have them; an older child might be helped by shots *if* it is definitely known that the asthma is a reaction to an allergen, *if* there is an effective antigen available, *if* strict and carefully observed avoidance tactics have not worked, and *if* medications have proved ineffectual.
4. If your child is severely and chronically afflicted with asthma, consider getting a home air compressor (Pulmo-Aid or Dura-Neb 2000), which is an especially effective way of delivering beta agonists or cromolyn (see above).
5. Take heart from the knowledge that asthma, because of the physiology that underlies the disease, improves as children grow older. While they do not get rid of the disease (the tendency for the airway smooth muscle to get spastic is still there), the airways enlarge, and the symptoms decline in severity and eventually fade away to the

point where they are no longer evident to you or the child. Being patient, knowledgeable, and doing the right things when they need doing will speed this process along.

6. You can probably reduce the frequency, severity, and costs of your child's asthma attacks materially by getting involved in a childhood Asthma Self-Management Program. There are half a dozen or so of these programs around, and they are increasingly being made available through HMOs, hospitals, your local American Lung Association branch, and the Asthma and Allergy Foundation of America. These programs offer instruction, useful strategies, and practice in a variety of skills and procedures, which, when followed faithfully, help to prevent or control asthma attacks. To be put in touch with these programs in your area, contact your American Lung Association branch, the allergy department of your HMO, or your child's physician.
7. If you need help with a problem or an answer to a question about asthma, the National Asthma Center in Denver, Colorado, has a toll-free number you can call. The number is 800–222–LUNG.

12.

Hay Fever (Allergic Rhinitis — Chronic Runny Nose)

Children, from birth on, are subject to runny noses. The main reason is upper respiratory infections — colds and allergies — although a few youngsters do have chronic runny noses for no discernible cause. When the runny nose is the result of an allergy the condition is called allergic rhinitis. Allergic rhinitis is usually a reaction to plant pollens and so is commonly known as hay fever. However, a large number of other airborne substances, including house dust, mold, chemicals, and dander from animals, provoke symptoms identical to those of hay fever. This condition is simply called perennial or year-long allergic rhinitis. From a medical standpoint, the terms "hay fever" and "allergic rhinitis" are synonymous.

INCIDENCE

Allergic rhinitis is the most common allergy; over 20 million Americans have it. The seasonal form (hay fever) is twice as prevalent as the perennial variety (allergic reactions to house dust, mold, etc.). In the first 10 years of life, boys are more likely to have allergic rhinitis than girls. If either parent has allergic rhinitis, their children are three to five times more likely to have allergic rhinitis than if the parents were free of the disease.

TABLE 11
Symptoms of Allergic Rhinitis or Hay Fever

1. Repetitive sneezing, worse in the morning
2. An itch in the palate, throat, or ears
3. Dark circles or allergic "shiners" under the eyes
4. Itchy, watery eyes
5. Nasal stuffiness
6. A thin, watery mucus discharge from the nose
7. Feeling a persistent need to scratch or wrinkle the nose
8. Recurrent and unexplained nosebleeds
9. Loss of the sense of taste

USUAL AGE OF ONSET

Allergic rhinitis develops after a period of sensitization has taken place; hay fever, with its intermittent seasonal exposure to pollens, usually does not show up until the age of four. Since the triggers of perennial allergic rhinitis are constantly in the environment, this form develops more quickly; its symptoms can appear as early as 18 months of age.

SYMPTOMS

Table 11 lists the major symptoms of allergic rhinitis. With either seasonal or perennial allergic rhinitis the telltale symptom is repetitive sneezing; the unfortunate victim may reel off one sneeze after another, up to 20 or more in a brief period. This incessant, violent sneezing can quickly make the diaphragm, chest, and abdominal muscles tender and painful.

CAUSES

Allergic rhinitis is brought on by airborne allergens. Plant pollens (microscopic grains of protein material important to plant reproduction) cause hay fever. Determining which one or ones are to blame is fairly easy and is tied to the pollenation cycle of a limited number and type of plants. Grasses usually pollenate only in the spring; trees pollenate in the late winter and early spring; weeds pollenate throughout the summer and into the fall. Thus, if your child's symptoms begin in the very early spring and last for a brief period of time, chances are that tree pollen is involved. Appendix E, a pollen map and guide, will help you pin down likely offenders in your area.

Perennial allergic rhinitis is caused by breathing in molds, house dust (often containing dust mites and cockroach particles), or animal danders, especially those of cats and horses. There are skin tests and newer blood tests available that will enable your doctor and you to identify the specific agent more exactly. The place, the role, and the procedures followed in allergy testing are covered in more detail in Chapter 2. When the causes of the allergy are not absolutely clear, skin testing is a routine step in identifying the agent or agents responsible for your child's allergic rhinitis.

SKIN TESTS

Respiratory infections in children are so common and near-chronic that there is an understandable tendency to regard them as allergic in origin and to launch an expensive (and, in the end, unproductive) series of skin tests to identify the presumed causal agents. Skin tests should always be preceded by a complete, careful history and a scrupulous physical examination, which may be all that is required to account for the stubborn symptoms. See Chapter 11 for more on skin testing.

FIRST AID AND HOME TREATMENT OF HAY FEVER

Assuming that the diagnosis is accurate and the cause of your child's allergic rhinitis is positively identified, first aid and home treatment is the next step. There are two components:

1. *Help your child avoid altogether or reduce exposure to the cause or causes of the symptoms.*

This can often be accomplished simply by installing air purification equipment in the bedroom and seeing to it that the child has as little contact with the allergens as can be managed. (For instance, if a pet is responsible for the condition, it should not have entry to the house and certainly not to the child's room; if pollen is the villain, keep the youngster inside and quiet on high-pollen-count days.) Chapter 6 presents strategies to follow to avoid and control airborne allergens.

Parents sometimes ask about the advisability and effectiveness of moving away from a particular locality to escape a particular pollen. Even if the economic and social costs are disregarded, this is still a risky business because the new location may have other vegetation that will trigger the allergic reaction. If the cause of the reaction is definitely known and the resources are available, relocating temporarily during the height of the pollen season sometimes helps.

TABLE 12
Treatment for Hay Fever Symptoms

TYPE OF SYMPTOMS	*TREATMENTS*	*COMMENTS*
Mild, seasonal	Establish and avoid cause	Allergy Finder (Figure 1, pages 14–15) may help
	Use over-the-counter antihistamines as necessary; e.g., Actifed, Chlortrimeton, Dimetapp or Seldane (by prescription only)	Be alert to possible side effects; beware of dangerous interactions with alcohol, other drugs; if asthma symptoms also present, beware of sedation; usually no activity limitation necessary
Mild, perennial (year-round)	Establish and avoid cause	See above
	Invoke any necessary environmental controls	Air purifiers or conditioners can help greatly; other meausres aimed at blocking out or minimizing exposure to allergens also extremely useful
	Use over-the-counter antihistamines as necessary	See above
	If symptoms stubborn and not helped by OTC remedies, ask physician for prescription for intranasal steroids or Nasalcrom	Must be taken at least a week before they will affect symptoms; establish and use only minimum effective dose; avoid activities or environments that intensify symptoms
Moderate to severe, seasonal or perennial	Establish and avoid cause	See above
	Invoke any necessary environmental controls	See above
	Use prescription medications if necessary	See above
	Get allergy shots	If allergen has been positively identified and if indicated
	Reduce exposure by limiting activities appropriately	

Joyce, who is nine and lives in Davenport, Iowa, has been miserable the past three summers. During August and September she suffered acutely from severe hay fever, which slipped into moderate asthma on occasion. Ragweed caused her distress. This year her family spent their vacation along the southern edge of Lake Superior. Instead of leaving in early August, Joyce and her mother stayed on at the lake until Davenport had its first frost, which usually marks the end of the ragweed season. This year it happened in early September. Joyce missed the first week of school, but she did not mind missing the hay fever, which she avoided completely this time.

2. *You should administer medication as necessary after seeing your doctor.*

Table 12 lists the common treatment approaches to mild to severe hay fever. Table 13 lists the medications available and the ages at which they may be safely administered. The treatment of hay fever is almost

TABLE 13
Medications for Allergic Rhinitis for Use at Given Ages

	AGE			
MEDICATIONS	*UNDER 2*	*2–6*	*6–12*	*OVER 12*
Over-the-counter				
Antihistamines				
Actifed	No	Yes	Yes	Yes
Chlortrimeton	No	Yes	Yes	Yes
Prescription				
Antihistamines				
Seldane	No	No	No	Yes
Ornade spansules	No	No	No	Yes
Intranasal steroids				
Beconase	No	No	No	Yes
Vancenase	No	No	No	Yes
Nasalide	No	No	Yes	Yes
Intranasal cromolyn sodium				
Nasalcrom	No	Yes	Yes	Yes
Intransal decongestants	DO NOT USE — SEE TEXT			
Afrin				
Neosynephrine				
4-Way				

always successful if done correctly and if the child takes the medicine as prescribed.

For mild, seasonal hay fever, *antihistamines* are the mainstay of treatment. They work by counteracting the histamine that is released when antigens (pollens, etc.) invade the respiratory system. They have several serious drawbacks; they have a pronounced sedative effect, making the user drowsy and torpid, they sometimes cause gastric upsets or complaints, and they often make children irritable or even hyperirritable. Seldane, a relatively new antihistamine, does not carry the sedative side effects, but its high cost puts it out of the economic reach of most families. Nonetheless, it does work in many people and is a valuable treatment, especially for students who cannot tolerate the terrible drowsiness produced by other antihistamines. For more severe or stubborn cases of allergic rhinitis, your physician may prescribe either intranasal synthetic steroids or intranasal cromolyn sodium (see below).

The management of hay fever depends on the age of the child and the length of the allergy season. For infants under two years of age, chronic runny noses are almost always due to colds. In the very young child it is more appropriate to establish the cause of the runny nose positively and then take whatever steps are necessary to manage and reduce its complications.

Allergic rhinitis begins to show up in the young child from age four to eight with the symptoms growing more severe over time as the sensitivity to the allergen increases. For children who have mild to moderate symptoms lasting no more than four to six weeks, the usual procedure is to prescribe antihistamines, forewarning the parents of their sedative side effects.

Where the symptoms are severe or prolonged, *intranasal steroids* (Beconase, Vancenase, or Nasalide) virtually always work; *if they do not, the diagnosis of allergic rhinitis may be wrong*. Intranasal steroids are not approved for children under six, although it is not uncommon for doctors to prescribe them for somewhat younger children who are severely allergic. Administered as a nasal spray, they carry a cortisone-like medication. There is hardly any absorption of the medication so that cortisone's side effects are avoided. Intranasal steroids are extremely effective; for children with severe hay fever they are almost always the preferred treatment and are far superior to anything else available. Intranasal steroids are *preventive* measures; to be maximally effective they must be started before symptoms appear and continued without fail during the allergy season.

We do not advocate the use of either oral steroids (such as pills) or injectable steroids (steroid "shots") for the treatment of allergic rhinitis. Several years ago, at the peak of allergy season, it was not uncommon to administer a five- or seven-day course of prednisone or another cortisone by mouth. This was before the days of intranasal steroids. It was also not uncommon for people to get injections of a long-acting steroid known as Celestone. Both of these are unnecessary and may be dangerous. The long-term use of steroids can cause osteoporosis, a condition that causes the bones to thin. They may induce cataracts in the eyes. They may bring about destruction of the hip joint, a disease known as aseptic necrosis. They may even increase the likelihood of contracting serious infections. Thus, for a problem as mild as hay fever, it is unnecessary to use oral or injectable steroids. On the other hand, intranasal steroids do not carry these side effects and, if used as prescribed, may be safely taken over a period of years. For many allergy sufferers, the use of these preparations has been a godsend.

Mark has suffered from severe hay fever all of his life. He grew up in western Pennsylvania and moved to southern California when he was 15 years old.

He is now 25 and, while he loves the California weather, he despises the spring. As soon as the grass starts to grow, as soon as people begin to mow their lawns, he starts sneezing, particularly on a windy day. Sometimes he sneezes 10 to 15 times in a row, having to hear a "God bless you" each time. He has tried almost every antihistamine without success. Finally, two months ago, his physician gave him a prescription for Beconase. The doctor told him that it was preventive. He would have to take two sprays in each nostril twice a day, but he would not feel any different for five days. Five days later, his stuffy, scratchy, irritable nose and throat began to get better. A week after he began it, he could actually breathe for the first time in weeks. Two weeks later, it was as if he had no symptoms at all. He could not believe how much better he felt.

For the severely allergic child who gets side effects from intranasal steroids there is *intranasal cromolyn sodium* (Nasalcrom). Also a preventive measure, it has been available in the United States for several years. Administered as a nasal spray (a drop version is expected soon), it is effective in children as young as four years without causing irritation to their nasal membranes as intranasal steroids sometimes do, nor does it carry antihistamine's sedative side effects. Nasalcrom is generally not as effective as intranasal steroids. Sometimes these two types of sprays can both be used for severely allergic or otherwise nonresponsive youngsters.

There is a special word that must be said about decongestants. Decongestants are widely used in over-the-counter medications and are found in most cold medicines. By far the most common ingredient is pseudoephedrine, commonly known as Sudafed. It is unclear why these drugs have continued to enjoy such popularity. Probably it is because they have been around so long that no one has bothered to really examine them in detail. Almost all of them are available over-the-counter. There is no convincing evidence that the oral medications work; decongestant nasal sprays like Afrin and 4-Way among many others carry unpleasant side effects.

The use of these sprays may temporarily reduce the swelling in the nose and make your child feel better momentarily. However, after using one or another of them for more than a few days at a time, the nose actually becomes addicted to it. A disease known as *rhinitis medicamentosa* develops. This leads to swelling and clogging of the nasal membranes called turbinates. The swelling can be so bad that the child is unable to breathe and uses even more nasal spray. In time the child may be taking nasal spray 20 or more times a day.

Rhinitis medicamentosa is a disease that can be even more serious than hay fever. Treating this problem requires that the decongestants be stopped. In the first stages and in mild cases, the doctor would prescribe the intranasal steroids we discussed above. In more serious cases, a more potent intranasal spray known as Decadron Turbinaire would probably be called in. Decadron Turbinaire was widely used as an intranasal steroid before the days of Beconase and Vancenase. However, it can be absorbed by the body and can carry some of the same side effects as cortisone taken by mouth. Accordingly, except for this condition, it is very rarely used. For the most stubborn cases, it may be necessary to give cortisone by mouth for several days or longer to allow the nasal membranes to shrink. After they have shrunk, intranasal steroids can be begun. Rhinitis medicamentosa can be a very unpleasant disease to have and is often extremely difficult to treat. Accordingly, shun using intranasal decongestants in treating your child's nasal problems.

LONG-TERM TREATMENT

Long-term treatment of allergic rhinitis has three elements:

1. Constant, unrelenting avoidance or control of the triggers that precipitate attacks. This is the most important precaution you can take and one that you must impress on your child.
2. Appropriate use of medication.
3. Where indicated, desensitization (allergy shots).

In children whose symptoms persist for longer periods or are year-round, allergy shots may be effective. We strongly believe that only allergists should give or prescribe allergy shots, although there are many nonallergists who administer them. If you live in an area where one is available, we urge you to consult with or get a second opinion from a board-certified allergist.

Jill has had a chronic runny nose for the past four years. Her mother took her to Dr. Honald, a well-regarded ear, nose, and throat specialist who does some allergy on the side. He has not taken an allergy course in many years and, like many physicians, has not kept current with the recent developments in immunology. He treated Jill with allergy shots for her chronic runny nose. Her nasal symptoms improved with the shots, but, as her mother noted, her eczema, which had been mild, worsened. Dr. Honald did not believe that the symptoms were related but, at the mother's insistence, referred the child to an allergist. The allergist knew that allergy shots in children with eczema can make the skin get worse. She stopped the shots, prescribing intranasal steroids instead. The nasal symptoms cleared up. So did Jill's skin after the shots were stopped.

COMPLICATIONS

Runny noses result from a number of conditions, which can lead to a misdiagnosis of allergic rhinitis. *Upper respiratory infections (colds)* are sometimes difficult to distinguish from allergic rhinitis, although an infection is usually at fault if

1. Fever is present;
2. The nasal discharge is thick, yellow, or puslike; and
3. The mucus tissue has a characteristic boggy appearance.

Colds are often mistaken for allergies because colds are so prevalent in small children. Many parents complain that their preschoolers have runny noses all of the time, and the near-chronic infection can lead to the false conclusion that an allergy is to blame. In young children colds are especially problematic when child day care centers are in the picture or older children bring colds home. Chapters 5 and 20 tell you how you can decrease exposure to and minimize the severity of respiratory infections.

Vasomotor rhinitis sometimes occurs in children. With this condition, the blood vessels in the nose are nonspecifically reactive to irritants, and the nose gets inflamed and drippy for virtually any reason — cold weather, exercise, even eating hot soup. A careful examination by your doctor can usually establish that it is vasomotor rhinitis and not the result of an allergy.

Ear infections often accompany and are triggered by allergic rhinitis. See Chapter 16 for more about this common and troublesome condition.

Sinusitis is another fellow traveler of nasal allergies or infections. The sinuses are cavities located behind the nose and below the eyes. While their exact function is not clear, they are lined by the same tissue that lines the nose, and they open into the nose by small openings known as sinus ostia, normally allowing change of secretion produced in the sinuses. Anything that clogs the nose can block the sinuses and the inflammation called sinusitis can result. Rare in children under three years of age, it produces a variety of complaints — headaches, fever, a stuffy feeling at the back of the nose and under the eyes.

In children over three, sinusitis may be a chronic and often undiagnosed problem. It can only be confidently diagnosed with a sinus X ray. (While we do *not* advocate X rays be administered routinely, where chronic sinusitis is a possibility, an X ray should be done; a single picture can confirm the diagnosis of sinusitis and, if it is present, point to appropriate treatment.)

Runny noses result from a number of conditions, which can lead to a [illegible] cold or allergic [illegible]. [illegible] infants' colds are [illegible] difficult to distinguish from [illegible], although an infection is usually at fault if:

[illegible] is present.
The nasal discharge is thick [illegible] or pus-like, and [illegible]
The mucus is green or [illegible] appearance.

Colds are often mistaken for allergies because colds are so prevalent in small children. Many parents complain that their preschoolers have runny noses all of the time, and the near-chronic infection can lead to the [illegible] that an allergy is to blame. In young children colds [illegible] when day-care tenders are in the picture or older children bring colds home. Chapters 6 and 20 tell you how you can [illegible] exposure to and minimize the severity of respiratory infections.

[illegible] sometimes occurs in children. With this condition, the blood vessels of the nose are nonspecifically reactive to irritants, and the nose gets inflamed and drips for virtually any reason — cold weather, [illegible], even eating hot soup. A careful examination by your doctor can usually establish that it's [illegible] rhinitis and not the result of an allergy.

[illegible] infections often accompany and are triggered by allergic [illegible]. [illegible] the page about this [illegible] and troublesome condition. [illegible] is another [illegible] of nasal allergies or infections. The sinuses are cavities located behind the nose and below the eyes. While their exact function is not clear, they are lined by the same tissue that [illegible] the nose and drain into the nose through small openings known as [illegible], normally allowing drainage of secretion produced in the sinuses. Anything that clogs the nose can block the [illegible] and [illegible] a condition called sinusitis, [illegible] in children under three [illegible] indicates a variety of complaints — [illegible], fever, and [illegible] the back of the nose and under the eyes.

[illegible] over three months may be a chronic and often [illegible] condition. It can only be conclusively diagnosed with a sinus X-ray. [illegible] X-rays [illegible] and [illegible] should be done to [illegible] the diagnosis of sinusitis and, if it is present, point to appropriate treatment.

13.

Eczema and Dry Skin

Even though we are told that "beauty is only skin deep," our society so values clear, flawless skin that billions of dollars are spent each year on the hundreds of skin lotions, creams, cleansers, conditioners, and cover-ups that crowd drugstore shelves. Because of this attitude, skin problems — including those resulting from allergic skin disorders — cause considerable grief, much of which is avoidable.

The skin is an amazingly resilient organ. Left alone, or given the right kind of help, it often recovers completely from the most severe damage. This is especially true for allergic skin disorders whose lesions almost always clear up without a trace.

INCIDENCE

Eczema affects about 4 children in 100. It is slightly more common in girls but occurs equally often in the various racial or ethnic groups in the United States. It is more prevalent in urban, industrialized localities. If either parent has a history of hay fever, asthma, or eczema, the probability of eczema in the child increases substantially.

Dry skin (which is usually observed in children with eczema, although the reverse is not true) is a minor but annoying condition that can generally be managed without incident by following the procedures listed in Table 15.

TABLE 14
Classification of Eczema

STAGE	*TYPE OF LESION*	*USUAL SITES OF LESION*	*OTHER ASSOCIATED SYMPTOMS*
Infant (2 months–2 years)	Dry, chapped skin, which gives way to red, inflamed areas made up of small blisters; scratching leads to crusting and oozing	Cheeks, spreading to forehead, scalp, ears, trunk, and extremities	Irritability and sleeplessness
Childhood (2–12 years)	Red, inflamed areas of small blisters enlarged and encrusted by scratching; drier than in infant stage	Inside elbows and backs of knees; earlobes and behind ears	Dry skin, anxiousness, irritability, and hyperactivity
Adolescent and adult (over 12 years)	Large, thickened areas of skin surrounded by crusted blisters	Insides of elbows and knees, eyelids, wrists, hands, feet	Dry skin, prominent, profuse goosebumps

USUAL AGE OF ONSET

The majority of children with eczema develop it in infancy, somewhere between the second and twelfth month of life; approximately 90% of its victims turn up with the symptoms before they reach the age of five. The remaining 10% develop it in later childhood or even as adults.

SYMPTOMS

Regardless of the stage of life at which it turns up, eczema is accompanied by intense itching, which is its first, most prominent, and most distressing feature. The itching precedes the appearance of lesions, which take slightly different forms and blossom on different parts of the body, depending on the age at which they first appear. Table 14 classifies eczema according to age, type, and site of lesions, and other associated symptoms.

CAUSES

We do not definitely know the cause or causes of eczema. Onset or worsening of symptoms has been linked to some foods, to airborne allergens — pollens, house dust, molds, animal dander — and to psychological stress.

FOODS AND ECZEMA

Carefully conducted experiments using skin tests which tried to tie hypersensitivity to specific foods to eczema have proved inconclusive. In any case, routine skin testing for individuals suffering from eczema is not recommended because of the risk of triggering a reaction or worsening an existing one. Thus, all that can be said about eczema symptoms is that they are associated or linked with other bodily signs of allergy and are quite possibly made worse by exposure to allergy-producing substances to which the individual is susceptible — foods, dust and pollens, animal dander, molds. Consequently the sufferers or their parents must rely on elimination diets (see Chapter 4) or careful, critical observations to identify the agents that appear to produce or worsen the symptoms. Because of the possible role of foods in producing eczema, it is strongly recommended that newborn children with allergic parents be breast-fed for at least their first six months. This will delay the need to feed babies formula, milk, and other foods until later in the first year of life. Breast-fed babies, whether of allergic or non-allergic parents, have less eczema (indeed, fewer allergies of *all* kinds) than bottle-fed babies.

The treatment of eczema has to take into account a number of factors — type and extent of the disease, age and occupation of the victim, presence or absence of infection. The steps to follow in seeking help or relief are outlined below.

FIRST AID AND HOME TREATMENT OF ECZEMA

Home treatment of eczema has two aspects: controlling the itching and caring for the lesions. What you will do depends to some extent on the age of your child. Follow the steps in Table 15. In older sufferers with chronic, stubborn eczema, three to four brief exposures per week to ultraviolet light (sunlight) can relieve mild or moderate symptoms. Avoid sunburn!

Wes, a teenager, learned the hard way that too much sun can add up to disaster. He heard that psoriasis, another skin disease, is helped by sunlight. Accordingly he bought a sunlamp, used the protective glasses as advised, and gradually acclimated his skin to increasing exposure over a seven-day

TABLE 15
First Aid and Home Treatment for Eczema

1. *Check for infection.* If serious scratch marks, widespread lesions, significant crusting, or severe discoloration are present, SEE A PHYSICIAN TODAY. (Infections are common with eczema; antibiotics are the usual and effective means of treatment.)
2. *To Control itching, scratching, and spread of lesions*
   — Keep fingernails trimmed as short as possible.
   — Avoid activities causing excessive sweating or emotional stress.
   — DO NOT wear tight or overly warm clothing.
   — DO NOT wear wool or other harsh fabrics.
   — Avoid temperature extremes.
   — Avoid harsh soaps, detergents, and petrochemicals (Dove is recommended as a mild soap. DO NOT use Ivory as it is very irritating to eczema).
   — Apply protective dressings and, if necessary, protective cuffs in the case of infants and small children.
   — Apply Burow's solution to the "wet" type of lesion (Burow's solution, aluminum acetate, is available over-the-counter at the pharmacy. Follow directions for preparation and application strictly).
3. *If the foregoing remedies do not give relief, consult a physician.* The physician will likely prescribe corticosteroid creams or ointments, which are effective for control of spread of lesions, and antihistamines, which, probably because of their sedative effect, sometimes relieve itching and scratching.
4. *About bathing,* opinion is divided. We believe bathing where the "dry" type of eczema is involved should be limited to two or three times per week. Leisurely baths (30 minutes or more) in tepid water are recommended. Non-lanolin-based oils and non-irritating soaps such as Dove should be used. A lotion applied to the body after bathing soothes and relieves itching and prevents excessive drying of skin. Use non-water-based cleansers like Cetaphil between baths.
5. *Elimination diets,* which take account of suspected food irritants, should be instituted and followed strictly for at least two weeks (see Appendix A for detailed instructions).
6. *Other suspected irritants* should be controlled as much as possible (see Chapter 8 for advice).
7. *Allergy shots* are usually to be *avoided* because of the danger of provoking a reaction and because eczema does not respond especially well to this form of treatment.

period. By the week's end, he was using it one hour per day. Within two weeks, his skin was dry and itchy. After three weeks his skin was an inflamed mess.

LONG-TERM TREATMENT

If you follow the procedures covered in Table 15 faithfully, your child's eczema will usually respond to them. If the symptoms persist, get worse, or the lesions become infected, see your pediatrician or family practitioner *at once*. In addition, take steps to identify and avoid any substances that are associated with the appearance or worsening of symptoms. Foods (milk, eggs, wheat, legumes, fish, potatoes) and airborne antigens (pollens, mold, dust, animal dander) are the most common offenders (see Chapters 4 and 6). Skin tests can help to pin down the allergens associated with eczema but they should be used cautiously because they can trigger eczema symptoms.

Finally, try to create an atmosphere that is free of psychological stress for your child by concentrating on doing specific things to relieve the discomfort. Do not try to control scratching by nagging or punishing the child. Such actions will not relieve the fierce itching and may simply focus attention on the complaint rather than persuading or making it possible for the child to leave the itchy spots alone.

DURATION

In infants eczema usually clears up without complications or any damage to the skin by the time the child turns four. In older children and adolescents the symptoms may persist — in about one fifth of cases — into adulthood, but they become more localized and usually respond to medication. The lesions can be quite unsightly and the temptation to mask them with cosmetics should be avoided, since many cosmetics contain substances that actually bring on the symptoms or make them worse.

COMPLICATIONS

Infections: Eczema lesions, because of the nearly irresistible temptation to scratch them, often develop secondary infections. Infections are usually treated with and respond to antibiotics, although antibiotic salves containing neomycin should be avoided in treating secondary infections of eczema.

Herpes simplex (fever blisters, cold sores): A herpes infection in a person with eczema can spread rapidly to cover much of the body and presents a serious threat. If eczema is accompanied or followed by a herpes infection, see your doctor immediately.

SPECIAL HINTS

While eczema lesions are unsightly they are not "catching," and you need not fear body contact with a child with eczema. It is perfectly safe for people with eczema to prepare or handle food and to have ordinary forms of contact with others.

Efamol (oil of evening primrose) is often recommended for treatment of eczema. The evidence indicates that it is not particularly effective with young children but in adolescents and adults it does help. It has two drawbacks; first, it is quite expensive. Second, over-the-counter imitations of Efamol, which are available in health food stores, differ chemically from the prescription version and their effectiveness has not been proved.

14.

Hives

INCIDENCE

Hives, known medically as urticaria, is the most common allergic or hypersensitivity reaction found in children. One person in five will have hives at one time or another.

USUAL AGE OF ONSET

Hives can crop up at any age. Children are especially likely to develop hives after eating certain foods or in conjunction with viral infections.

SYMPTOMS

Hives are blotchy patches of red, slightly elevated skin (wheals) which blanch or whiten when touched. The lesions, which can range in size from quite small to several inches in diameter, may cover much of the body in severe cases. They are usually intensely itchy, especially when located in areas covered by hair or in the webs of toes and fingers.

The *acute* form of the disorder follows release of histamine by the body's mast cells. This release of histamine may trigger a variety of reactions, one of which is the hive lesions.

Onset of the acute form of hives may be dramatically swift, with symptoms showing within minutes of exposure to a causal agent. Because of this narrow time gap between exposure and display of symptoms, it is often possible to make a hard and fast identification of the substance causing the outbreak.

The original wheals fade rapidly, ordinarily within the space of a few hours, but they also tend to migrate, relocating on other parts of the body. Where there is no additional exposure the symptoms customarily clear within a day or two, and they rarely persist for more than a week.

CAUSES

Often the symptoms so closely follow exposure to a trigger that the cause is obvious.

> Dan, 12, goes to a neighborhood park with a group of his friends for a game of touch football. During the course of the contest he takes off his shoes to improve his footing and, not long after that, steps on a bee which stings him. Within a few minutes, he develops a mild case of hives, intensely itchy wheals on his legs and in the groin area. By this time the foot that has been stung has swollen to the point where he is unable to put his shoe back on so he has to hobble home barefoot. When he gets home his father calls the doctor who tells them what to do to counter the pain, swelling, and itching and also informs them that this sort of reaction to a bee sting has serious implications. He says that Dan should be kept under observation for an hour or so and brought in to the office soon for a consultation. Dan's hives fade quickly and by the next morning he is clear of them, although the site of the bee sting is still tender and quite itchy.

Table 16 names the types of agents that most often provoke hives in children and lists a few of the many specific substances or conditions that produce them. There are also several special physical causes of hives or urticaria, which are described in Table 17.

Hives may show up as part of a more general or systemic reaction with anaphylactic shock a possibility. *Consequently, the appearance of hives should act as a signal to watch closely for the appearance of other possibly lethal signs.*

In the acute form the lesions usually clear up without incident in a day or two; if they persist for more than six weeks the condition is termed *chronic.* What provokes the chronic form of the complaint is much more difficult to establish, since histamine release does not seem to play a role. As a consequence, the search for the precipitating cause may be long, difficult, and, in about 70–80% of cases, unsuccessful.

Hives can also be associated with a number of chronic diseases including hyperthyroidism, systemic lupus erythematosus, juvenile

TABLE 16
Triggers for Hives in Children

CATEGORY	*PRINCIPAL OFFENDERS*
Food	Eggs, peanuts, nuts, chocolate, berries, seafood, tomatoes, milk, cheese, yeast
Food additives	Tartrazine, benzoates
Drugs	Penicillin, aspirin, and sulfonamides especially; almost all other drugs possible
Insects	Bites, stings, body material
Inhalants (rarely)	Pollens, dust, mold, animal dander
Infections	Viral infections, parasitic infestations, hepatitis, abscessed teeth
Systemic disease	Rheumatic disorders, hyperthyroidism, certain malignancies
Psychological factors	Extremes of tension, stress, anxiety

TABLE 17 Physical Urticarias — Recognition, Avoidance, and Treatment

NAME	*SYMPTOMS AND CAUSES**	*AVOIDANCE OR CONTROL STRATEGIES*	*TREATMENT*
Dermographism	Wheals in response to firm stroking of the skin	—	Antihistamines (Atarax)
Pressure urticaria	Red, deep, local painful swelling sometime after skin is exposed to sustained pressure (as of shoes, belts, etc.)	Relieve pressure	*Does not* respond to antihistamine. Low dosage of prednisone helpful
Cold-induced urticaria	Burny, itchy eruption, headache, wheezing, fainting within minutes of exposure to cold	Dress warmly, warm gradually	Desensitize to prevent wheezing triggered by exposure to cold. A drug called Periactin is often very effective
Heat-induced urticaria	Wheals after contact with heated object or hot bath or shower	Avoid heat	Antihistamines (if necessary)
Cholinergic urticaria	Small wheals (1–2mm) surrounded by larger inflamed red patches associated with elevated core body temperature (i.e., following exercise, bathing)	Take medication before exercise	Antihistamines (Atarax)
Solar urticaria	Itchy red patches within minutes of exposure to sun or artificial light	Use a sunscreen	Antihistamines

*This table lists only the most common causes of physical urticaria in children. There are many other substances or factors known or thought to trigger hives, although they are rarely encountered in practice.

rheumatoid arthritis, lymphoma, and some cancers. As with most other allergic reactions, the underlying causes or mechanisms that produce hives remain unknown.

TREATMENT OF HIVES

While hives usually vanish after a short period of time, leaving only the memory of blemishes and acute discomfort from the itching, they should be watched closely for two reasons:

1. They may be associated with serious or even life-threatening complications that require drastic emergency treatment.
2. They sometimes accompany chronic noninfectious diseases. Skin testing and courses of allergy shots are generally not recommended for treatment of hives. The mainstay of treatment is the use of antihistamines to reduce itching. Sadly, while antihistamines are often effective, they almost always induce severe sedation. If you use antihistamines other than Seldane, be very careful of this side effect. Do not drive or operate machinery.

Lauren could predict her school grades by the amount of antihistamines she took. The higher the dose, the worse her exam scores. Fortunately, her doctor found out that Lauren's hives could be controlled by Seldane, an antihistamine that does not cause sedation.

First-aid and home-treatment measures for hives appear in Table 18.

LONG-TERM TREATMENT

Acute hives rarely persist for more than a few days. If they hang on for longer than 48 hours of if they resist treatment, see your doctor. The doctor may try different types of antihistamines from the mild OTC drugs such as Chlortrimeton to potent very sedative-inducing drugs such as Benadryl, Atarax, and Vistaril. On occasion, tranquilizers such as Sinequan may be used. While Sinequan does have antianxiety properties, it is an extremely potent antihistamine. Control of anxiety can also help reduce the itching and therefore, the hives. Thus, Sinequan is often effective. However, there is little evidence that hives are psychologically induced.

For very severe cases of chronic hives, your doctor may also prescribe Cimetidine, a drug that has generally been used to treat the acidity associated with ulcers. Finally, for chronic relentless cases, steroids may

TABLE 18
First Aid and Home Treatment for Hives (Acute type with sudden onset)

1. *Take oral antihistamines* (Benadryl, Chlortrimeton, Dimetane, Atarax) for lesions and relief of itching.
2. *Keep victim quiet for at least 30 minutes* and watch closely for additional reactions. ANY OF THE FOLLOWING, IF THEY APPEAR, REQUIRE THAT THE INDIVIDUAL RECEIVE EMERGENCY MEDICAL TREATMENT AT ONCE. IF NECESSARY, SUMMON FIRE DEPARTMENT, RESCUE SQUAD, OR AMBULANCE.
   — difficulty with breathing
   — abdominal pain
   — difficulty in swallowing
   — weakness
   — confusion
   — bluish or purplish coloration
   — irregular or thready pulse
   — incontinence
   — constricted feeling in chest
   — wheezing
   — nausea or vomiting
   — hoarseness or thickened speech
   — drop in blood pressure
   — collapse
   — unconsciousness
3. *If hives alone worsen or persist for more than 48 hours,* see a physician as soon as possible. (The physician will take a history and may order laboratory tests to try to pinpoint causes and, *most important,* rule out the possibility that other, more serious diseases or infections are responsible for the reaction.)
4. *Avoid* vasodilators including alcohol, aspirin, heat, exertion, and emotional stress.
5. *Avoid* quinine, opiates (codeine, meperidine, morphine), antibiotics (chlortetracycline, polymyxins), and certain vitamins (thiamine), which can directly release allergic mediators from mast cells.
6. *To control itching* (additional measures)
   — take tepid water baths to which Aveeno colloidal oatmeal has been added.
   — apply cool or ice compresses.
   — use itch-suppressing lotions such as 0.25% menthol ± 1% phenol in calamine lotion (Eucerin), Schamberg's lotion, or Caladryl.
7. It is *rarely* necessary to use cortisone in the treatment of hives, although it is sometimes helpful for severe *acute* urticaria, pressure urticaria, or urticaria associated with systemic lupus erythematosus.

be used, although we try to avoid them whenever possible because of their serious side effects (see Chapter 12, page 106).

ANGIOEDEMA

Angioedema, which is often associated with hives, may occur as single or multiple and widespread lesions. Unlike hives, however, its nonpitting, sharply demarcated, and *nonitching* swellings may crop up at any place on or in the body. Lesions of angioedema, like those of hives, may be of short duration, but if they do persist they migrate every 24 to 48 hours. In angioedema (*angio* — blood; *edema* — swelling) the soft tissues around the eyes, the lips, and the genitals are often involved, and the gastrointestinal and pulmonary tracts may be affected. Swelling in the larynx which sometimes occurs is dangerous and, in rare instances, fatal, causing death by asphyxiation.

About 10% of the population may experience both hives and angioedema; hives alone will be seen in 8% and angioedema alone will affect

2% of the population. For unknown reasons angioedema occurs more frequently in women 40 to 49 years of age; it is uncommon in children.

In almost three quarters of cases the precipitating cause of angioedema is unknown. Moreover there is no reliable way to diagnose angioedema with laboratory tests. One exception to this statement is a rare familial angioedema known as hereditary angioneurotic edema. (The allergist is often in the awkward position of having to say, "You've got so-and-so but I can't tell you what's causing it." This is especially true for angioedema.)

There are good reasons for getting a confirmed diagnosis of angioedema. First, the disorder comes in two forms, one acquired and one inherited or genetically transmitted. Individuals having *hereditary* angioedema can be treated medically so as to minimize the risk and the severity of attacks.

Second, in either its hereditary or acquired form, angioedema is potentially life-threatening, and individuals having the disorder should be aware of its existence. They should also know what steps to take in the event of an attack and wear Medic-Alert identification so that others will also know of and be able to respond swiftly and appropriately in an emergency.

Attacks of angioedema have been associated with the following conditions:

- Trauma or injury (especially to soft tissue of the upper respiratory tract such as occurs in tooth extraction or tonsillectomy)
- Heavy exposure to inhalant allergens (dusts or pollens)
- Strenuous exercise
- Cold
- Vibration
- Pressure

First aid and home treatment for children diagnosed as susceptible to angioedema are given in Table 19.

TABLE 19
First Aid and Home Treatment for Angioedema

1. If red, raised, *nonitching* lesions on the surface of the skin are present, *administer antihistamines* such as Benadryl or Atarax.
2. If mucus or soft tissue is affected, *watch closely for additional symptoms.* IF ANY OF THE FOLLOWING APPEAR, SEEK EMERGENCY MEDICAL TREATMENT AT ONCE. IF NECESSARY, SUMMON FIRE DEPARTMENT, RESCUE SQUAD, OR AMBULANCE.
   — difficulty with breathing
   — difficulty in swallowing
   — abdominal pain
   — constricted feeling in throat or chest
   — hoarseness or thickened speech

After initial attack

3. *See a physician (allergist) as soon as possible* for diagnostic tests and medical treatment of the herditary form of the disorder if it is found, or medical control of the acquired form.
4. *Avoid any known precipitating causes.*
5. *Avoid the following possible precipitating causes:*
   — trauma or physical injury
   — dusts and pollens
   — strenuous, taxing exercise
   — extremes of cold
   — vibration
   — pressure
6. *Carry and know how to use a kit for anaphylactic emergencies* (GET A PRESCRIPTION FOR AN ANA-KIT FROM YOUR DOCTOR).
7. *Wear a Medic-Alert bracelet, appropriately inscribed* (see Chapter 9, page 66, for address of the Medic-Alert Foundation).

15.

Itchy Eyes

Everyone, at some time or another, has probably had red, itchy eyes. A child can get itchy eyes from scores of things. Dirt and foreign material or objects in the eye are most commonly responsible. Yet, few people realize the large number of causes of red eyes. Here are accounts of four children who were taken to allergists because of suspected allergies. All had similar symptoms but vastly different diagnoses.

Bob, 11, plays left field for his Little League baseball team. No matter what he seems to do his eyes get red during games. His mother is convinced that he is allergic to his baseball glove. His doctor is convinced there is nothing wrong with him. His father is convinced that it is all in his head. Bob knows it gets worse during the daytime, whenever he looks into the sun, and especially when he is out there in the field, staring intently, waiting for a ball to be hit to him. As it happens, Bob's eyes are simply very sensitive to sunlight, which causes them to water copiously. As they water, Bob rubs them to clear his vision. The process of rubbing produces a simple nonallergic irritation. A pair of sunglasses was all he needed to clear up the problem.

Doe, 13, is taken to her doctor because she has severely swollen, red, and itchy eyelids. Her mother is convinced her problems are from using eye makeup. In this case Mom has it right. Doe is allergic to some of the chemicals in the makeup which are very irritating to her tender skin.

Paul, 12, gets severely itchy eyes every spring — they become so swollen that he can barely see. He often has chronic repetitive sneezing at the same time. His eyes almost always get worse on a windy day or when the meteorologist says the pollen count is high. Paul has classic hay fever and allergic conjunctivitis. His treatment, avoidance and eye drops, is extremely effective.

Charley's dad is a house painter who carries all of his materials — paints, brushes, turpentine, ladders, etc. — in the back of the family van. Charley's eyes begin to water as soon as he gets in the vehicle. His dad thought it was due to an allergy to the vinyl upholstery. He could not believe it could be from the paint and the fumes because Charley, 10, had been riding in the van for years without any problem. Nonetheless, problems, habits, and irritations change, and his son's watery eyes are in fact due to fumes.

Doe and Paul's are allergic reactions; Bob and Charley's are simple irritations.

INCIDENCE

Allergic conjunctivitis, chronically red and itching eyes, is a common problem in children. It usually accompanies hay fever.

USUAL AGE OF ONSET

Allergic conjunctivitis usually shows up in four- to six-year-olds, although it may appear at any age thereafter. If your child has never had any allergies and then begins to develop eye symptoms after age 16, the symptoms are probably not allergic, although, as in everything else in life, there are some exceptions.

Kevin, now 17, lived in Detroit, Michigan, until last year when his family moved to Dodge City, Kansas. Kevin had no allergies in Detroit but within the first year after settling in Dodge City, began to complain that his eyes and his ears itched. Also, he noticed that in the morning he sneezed uncontrollably seven or eight times in a row. His parents couldn't understand why, out of the blue, Kevin suddenly developed allergies. What they didn't realize is that Kevin had moved out of the cement city into farm — and pollen — country.

SYMPTOMS

Allergic conjunctivitis is usually bilateral, that is, it involves both eyes. They will be red and itchy and will worsen with rubbing. The itching and inflammation will vary in intensity with location. They will usually be worse out-of-doors if the offending agent is pollen, or indoors if the offending agent is house dust or animal dander.

If the child has involvement in only one eye, BEWARE! This might be a severe infection.

The irritation, if it is due to allergies, will virtually always appear about the same time as other allergies, particularly hay fever, crop up. Thus, it is unusual to have allergic eyes without also having an allergic runny nose or asthma or some other allergic disease.

CAUSES

The causes of allergic conjunctivitis are the big five of allergies — tree pollen, grass pollen, weed pollen, house dust, and animal dander. Molds generally do not produce allergic conjunctivitis. By far the biggest offenders are grass pollen and animal dander. Grass pollen is a major cause, simply because there is so much of it in the springtime and because children play out-of-doors and are exposed to it. Animal dander, equally problematic, is prevalent indoors; it occurs because it is so easy to get animal dander on the fingers and transfer it to the eyes. Children also develop symptoms from picking up animal dander inadvertently.

Brad, 9, has been visiting his grandma's house virtually every Sunday since he was an infant. His mother has always known that he is allergic to his grandma's dog, so she has him wash his hands thoroughly and cautions him not to rub his eyes whenever he is at Grandma's house. On a recent trip, the family put up at a motel in Oregon. Within 30 minutes of arriving in the room, Brad began to sneeze and to rub his eyes. His eyes were itching and tearing so badly that he was practically crying. His mother recognized his symptoms as being the same as the ones he got at Grandma's house. While there were no animals in the room she came to realize later that many travelers bring dogs and cats into motel rooms — and motel housekeeping is often so haphazard that the animal dander would pile up for succeeding guests.

WHEN TO SEE THE DOCTOR

The biggest problem with allergic conjunctivitis is not the allergy itself, but the tendency to confuse it with other eye problems. Serious bacterial infections of the eye often mimic allergic conjunctivitis, and only a good examination by the doctor will pick up the difference. *This is not an exam that you should do.* This is because certain *viral* infections can closely resemble bacterial infections or allergic symptoms and can be very severe. Adenovirus and herpes viruses, two frequent causes of eye irritation, are found everywhere on the body. All too often these viruses get in the child's eye. The parents may think an allergy is responsible because the viral symptoms closely resemble allergic ones. They respond by administering the same eye drops prescribed for allergic conjunctivitis. The trouble is that some of the eye drops designed to treat allergic conditions have steroids in them; when these steroids are put into an *infected* eye, the disease can virtually explode, even bringing about blindness.

Suzy, 11, has had allergic conjunctivitis for several years. The symptoms usually appear only during the months of May and June when the pollen count is high. However, in mid-November, not long after a cold, her mother noted that Suzy's eyes were quite red and teary. She assumed it was from her allergies and she put eye drops, containing steroids, in Suzy's eyes. These were the drops that the doctor had prescribed during springtime for Suzy. This time, Suzy had an adenovirus infection of her eyes and the eye drops caused a severe reaction. Fortunately, the medication did not bring about significant impairment in vision, although it could easily have led to scarring of the cornea and total loss of vision.

Unless the symptoms are unmistakably and clearly familiar and follow an established allergic pattern, *take all eye problems to your child's doctor*.

FIRST AID AND HOME TREATMENT OF ITCHY EYES

The *first* thing to do in allergic conjunctivitis is to establish the cause of the problem. Use the criteria and standards we have listed above to do this.

Second, identify the reason. Reviewing the questions in Figure 5, a good checklist of the potential triggers, will help you do this.

Third, impose environmental controls to the fullest extent possible (see Chapter 6 for methods of controlling airborne allergens). Keep fingers out of eyes. Scratching and rubbing the eyes will only make the symptoms worse.

Fourth, apply ocular antihistamines, prescription medications which contain the same antihistamines used to treat hay fever. These are very effective in reducing the itching and the redness of allergic conjunctivitis. Since they are put into eyes they do not produce the sedation that they do when taken by mouth, although they can cause irritation in some susceptible persons. Intraocular cromolyn, much like the cromolyn used for allergic rhinitis or asthma, is also available. While expensive and no more effective, it is less irritating than antihistamines and is used by many patients for long-term treatment. The medications used to treat allergic conjunctivitis and comments on their advantages and

FIGURE 5
Allergic Conjunctivitis Test Questions

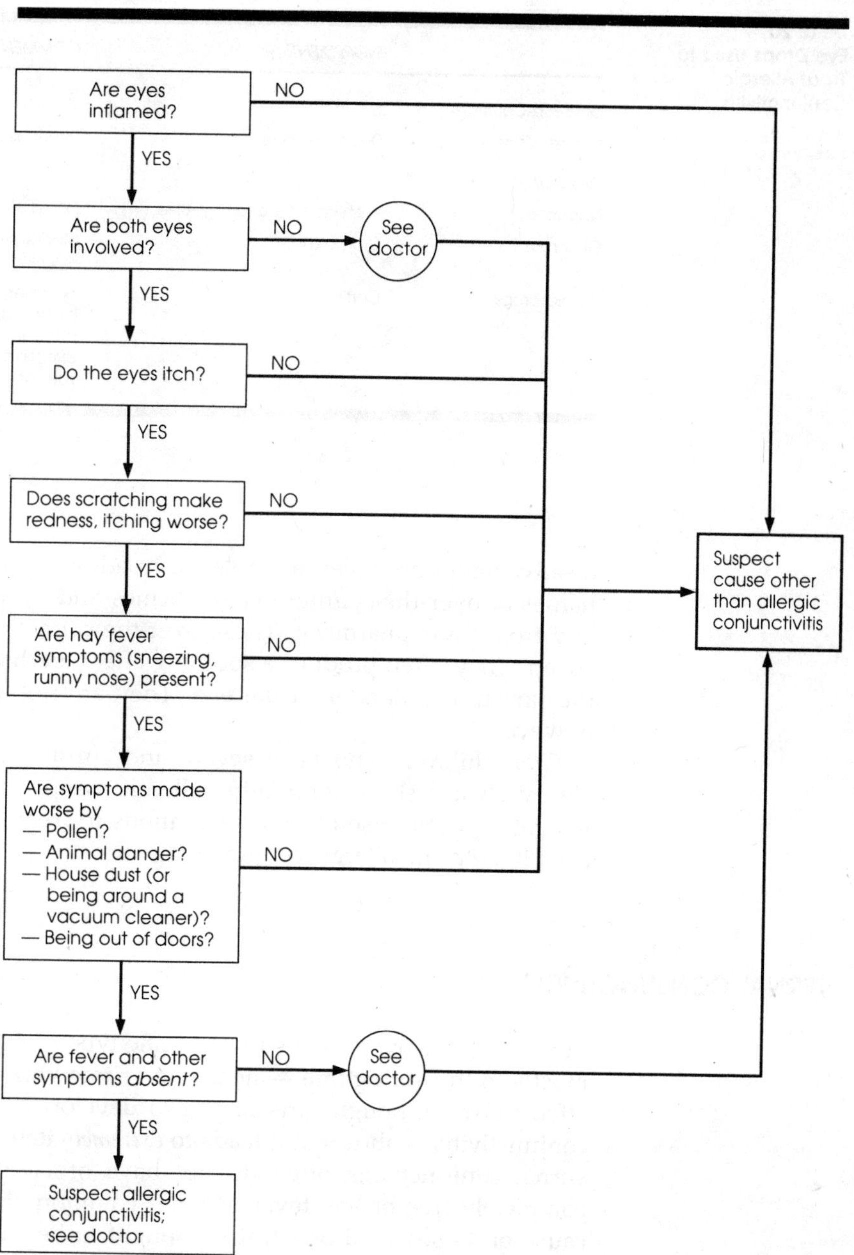

TABLE 20 Eye Drops Used to Treat Allergic Conjunctivitis

	INGREDIENTS	*COMMENT*
Over-the-Counter		
Murine, Visine	Decongestants	Reduces eye redness
Prescription		
Naphcon	Antihistamine decongestive	Extremely effective
Opticrom	Cromolyn	Moderately effective. Best drug for long-term usage
Steroid drops	Cortisone	Extremely effective; when used inappropriately, can cause dangerous complications or side effects; *any use* should be OK'd by your doctor

disadvantages are given in Table 20. In addition, Table 20 contains the names of over-the-counter eye medicines and eyewashes that you can buy from your pharmacy. These over-the-counter drugs are relatively cheap. They often produce a soothing effect, perhaps by flushing away the pollen and dander in the eye. They are not a long-term remedy, however.

Fifth, children who have severe and chronic allergic conjunctivitis almost always show some other allergic symptom, such as hay fever. Accordingly, the use of oral medications to treat these symptoms will usually help the allergic conjunctivitis too.

VERNAL CONJUNCTIVITIS

Vernal conjunctivitis refers to a specific type of eye irritation occurring mostly in the springtime — hence, the name vernal. Most commonly it affects boys although girls may also develop it. The onset of vernal conjunctivitis is abrupt and leads to *extremely* itchy eyes. Children with vernal conjunctivitis often do not have other allergies and may be completely free of hay fever or other common allergic symptoms. Because of its seasonal onset, it is thought to be allergic, but we do not know exactly what causes it. The best way to determine if your child has this condition is to have an examination by an allergist or an eye doctor. The doctor will invert the eyelid to look at its underside; where vernal conjunctivitis is involved the underside of the lid has a characteristic and unmistakable cobblestone appearance. Treatment calls for oral antihistamines, eye drops, and (very important) avoiding scratching the eyes. Fortunately, most children eventually grow out of this condition by the late teens.

CONTACT LENSES

A special form of eye irritation is seen in people who wear the newer plastic contact lenses. It is rare in young children (most of whom do not wear contacts) but is found in adolescents and certain young adults. Children — and adults — who do wear the new plastic contact lenses can develop a condition known as follicular hyperplasia. It results from inappropriate or incomplete cleansing of the contact lens. This may trigger an allergic response resulting in blurring of vision and significant irritation of the eyes. The best treatment for this condition is to avoid the cause — in other words, wear eyeglasses. Although many ophthalmologists allow patients to continue to wear their contacts when this condition develops, persisting with the contact lenses can prove harmful and damaging to the eyes.

EYE EXAMINATIONS

The eyes are a precious commodity and remind us of an important additional note. In some schools eye tests are administered to virtually every child every year, and if the exam is failed the child is referred to his or her doctor. In other places the exam may occur once every several years or not at all. Children doing badly in school are often referred to allergists. This happens because of the persistent misconception that obscure, undiagnosed allergies, even in otherwise healthy-appearing children, can impair their ability to learn. Sometimes we find the problem is nothing more than poor vision.

> Sean is an active and seemingly very bright eight-year-old who has great difficulty in reading. School officials thought his reading problem was due to allergies. It quickly became apparent to his allergist that he suffered from a condition known as dyslexia. Dyslexia, a complex but not uncommon perceptual problem, is not due to allergies. Sean simply got lost in the mass of students and managed to get by each year without receiving an accurate diagnosis *and* help. Sean was referred to a reading tutor in his district. Over the next several years he was able to make enormous progress.

CARE OF THE EYES

As a parent, make it a point to have your child's vision checked periodically; weak or defective eyesight can drastically lower school performance. Reading difficulties, like dyslexia, can be brought out by having your child read aloud to you. If there seems to be trouble recognizing simple words in context, consult with the child's teacher and the school's or district's reading specialist.

There is an old adage that warns, "Never put anything smaller than your elbow in your eye." The eyes are precious and nothing should be placed in them, medication or otherwise, without help and advice.

16.

Earache

Earaches in children are usually the result of an infection in the middle ear. *Otitis media,* the medical name for the condition, means exactly that.

Stacey's parents well remember her fourth birthday. She woke up that day cranky and irritable; her parents thought it might be due to excitement in anticipation of the day's activities. Stacey had a series of crying fits and temper tantrums and the party went badly. This behavior was unusual, and by evening her parents sensed that she might be ill. They took her temperature and, finding that it was 101.5, gave her some liquid Tylenol which brought the fever down and quieted her. At two o'clock in the morning Stacey awakened, screaming and crying uncontrollably. She complained that her ears hurt. Her temperature was 103.5 and she could not be comforted. Her dad, frantic, bundled her up and took her to the emergency room at the local hospital where the doctor examined her ears and said that she had a bulging eardrum, characteristic of acute otitis media. Stacey's parents had never heard of otitis media but quickly learned how common chronic infected ears can be. Stacey was given a decongestant, an antibiotic, and some medicine for her fever. Within a few hours she felt better and her temperature quickly returned to normal. Over the next year, though, Stacey had five more of these episodes. Her parents thought an allergy might be responsible and took the child to an allergist. The allergist took a careful history and quickly concluded that this was all a by-product of colds and the unique anatomy of children's eustachian tubes and ear canals. No allergy was implicated in her case.

INCIDENCE

As near as we can judge, about one half of all children have an earache at least once; chronic, recurrent earaches are among the more frequently encountered problems in the pediatrician's office. Boys, obese children, and allergic children (or children of allergic parents) tend to be more susceptible to earaches.

USUAL AGE OF ONSET

Earache due to infection is a childhood disease and is mainly seen in infants, toddlers, and especially preschoolers. It becomes increasingly less prevalent in older age groups and rarely shows in adolescents or adults. This age-related drop in prevalence of symptoms is a direct result of maturation and the physiological changes that accompany it.

SYMPTOMS

The symptoms of an earache are not directly observable by you, the parent. Indeed, they are likely to show up in children too young to tell you exactly how they feel. What you observe in the behavior and appearance of the child tells you or makes you suspect an ear infection, either acute or chronic. An acute ear infection can make its presence known in a variety of ways:

- Tugging of the earlobe
- Excruciating pain accompanied by severe distress, restlessness
- Fever, sometimes quite high (103.5+)

Chronic ear infections are implicated in

- Persistent mild, dull earache
- Sense of fullness or stuffiness in the head ("My head feels funny")
- Popping sensation in the ears, as occurs during rapid changes in elevation
- Low-grade fever

Temporary or permanent hearing loss is a common and serious aspect of acute or chronic ear infections in children. Indications of hearing loss are subtle and develop almost imperceptibly. Be alert to the following signs of hearing impairment in your youngsters, especially if there are recurrent bouts of earache.

- Inattentiveness, slowness in attending or responding to others, disobedience
- Need for you to speak loudly or to repeat what you have said in order to be understood
- In school-age children, underachievement, withdrawal

There are also a few physical tip-offs to the possibility of ear infection.

- In infants or young children, incessant tugging or clawing at the ear
- Allergic "shiners" — dark shadows under the eyes
- Mouth breathing. This suggests that the nose is chronically stuffed and, possibly, the ear blocked as well (Mouth breathers often complain of a bad morning taste in the mouth, this because the mouth is dried out from the passage of air through it rather than the nose.)

CAUSES

Earaches result from a structural, anatomical flaw in children. The eustachian tube, a short, slender pipe that connects ear and nose, is much smaller in diameter, runs more horizontally, and has a thicker lining of mucus tissue in children than it does in adults. When an upper respiratory infection (colds or flu) hits or when nasal allergies (hay fever; perennial allergic rhinitis — see Chapter 12) show up, the eustachian tube can get clogged and inflamed. All debris in the tube becomes trapped inside; a bacterial infection then develops in the middle ear and exerts pressure on the ear drum. Pain and the other symptoms described above follow.

The blockage of the immature eustachian tube results most often from viral colds and allergies, generally with a secondary bacterial infection. However, there are other causes as well, including colds, allergies, enlarged adenoids, foreign objects, cleft palate, injuries, and, rarely, nasopharyngeal cancer.

WHEN TO SEE THE DOCTOR

Because of the extreme pain and discomfort involved and the distinct threat of hearing impairment that chronic, untreated ear infections present, you should consult your doctor at the first sign of an earache. An untreated earache, if due to a bacterial infection, can even lead to meningitis and death.

If your child is allergic, any examination of the child in connection with the allergic condition should always include a look into the ears.

If the doctor overlooks this important step, offer a gentle reminder to carry it out. ("Wouldn't you like to examine the ears, too?")

FIRST AID AND HOME TREATMENT OF EARACHE

For the child who is susceptible to ear infections, the first and most effective line of treatment is prevention. Where the earaches are allergy-related (and they will be allergy-related *only* if allergic symptoms like hay fever or asthma are also present), identify and avoid the agent responsible. (See Chapter 6 for information on how to avoid or control airborne allergens.) Where the earaches are due to respiratory infections, follow the procedures given in Chapters 5 and 20 to reduce exposure to and control colds and coughs.

In addition, in infants, *avoid* the use of pacifiers, poorly vented nursing bottle nipples, feeding the baby when it is supine, and bottle-propping (for self-feeding), as all of these practices can result in aspiration of fluid into the middle ear and eventual infection. You may also want to consider humidifying the sleeping room (see Chapter 20 for suggestions about humidifiers) to help keep the respiratory membranes moist and functioning effectively.

Treatment for earache is ordinarily doctor-initiated; *folk remedies are ineffectual*. Where an allergy is responsible a prescription antihistamine decongestant is usually administered. If bacterial infection is also present, an antibiotic will be prescribed. This ordinarily clears up the infection rapidly.

Carefully follow the physician's and pharmacist's instructions about frequency and duration of administration of medications. Neglecting to do this — stopping antibiotics too soon, for example — can result in a quick and stubborn rebound of the infection. Insist on getting information on any medications prescribed, and be alert to possible side effects. If side effects develop, notify your physician at once.

Finally, *DO NOT* probe or attempt to put anything into the ear. This practice can cause serious damage to the delicate structures in the ear and may result in injury and hearing loss.

LONG-TERM TREATMENT

If your young child develops acute ear infections several times per year you should seriously consider having ear tubes implanted. These are plastic inserts which are put in the ears by an ear, nose, and throat specialist. The plastic tubes help drain and ventilate the ear canal, thereby reducing the risk of developing recurrent infections. It is a minor surgical procedure performed on an outpatient basis and often proves extremely helpful. In addition, when the tubes are implanted the physician has the opportunity to remove any fluid or debris that has remained trapped behind the eardrums. This removal of fluid acts to prevent further infection or even hearing loss.

Ear tubes do carry some disadvantages you ought to know about:

- In very young children they have a tendency to fall out. This is troublesome although essentially harmless.
- Children with ear tube implants must either use earplugs or exercise extreme care to avoid getting water into their ears while bathing. Swimming or showering should be avoided.

Ear tubes are not for everyone and work best for younger children with recurrent problems that are not rapidly responsive to antibiotics. We should also note that the effectiveness of ear tubes has recently been questioned. In our experience, they work best for young children (less than six years old) who have more than four ear infections per year. Moreover, if your child responds rapidly to antibiotics (within 24 hours) the ear tubes are probably not needed.

COMPLICATIONS OF EARACHES

Hearing loss, temporary or permanent, is a common companion of ear infections.

> Holly, who is 11, is an excellent reader, but she seems not to follow verbal directions very well. While she is a pleasant and attractive youngster, she is often seen playing alone, in and out of school. She was referred to an allergist because her school performance seemed far below her potential, as evidenced by her test scores. As part of the exam, the allergist looked in her ears. The eardrums appeared normal but her tympanogram was abnormal. A tympanogram is a test that measures the ability of the eardrum to retract. The doctor wondered whether she had a gluey ear from chronic untreated ear infections, so he referred her to an audiologist. The audiologist found that Holly had a minor but significant hearing deficit and prescribed a hearing aid. This helped her enormously. When the device was installed, Holly's immediate reaction was to ask, *"Why is everybody shouting?"* But Holly adapted to it quickly and, while her hearing is not completely normal, her parents and teachers are amazed at how much her school performance and her social relationships have improved.

You can crudely assess the possibility of a hearing loss in your child by using a watch — one that ticks, of course. In a quiet room with the child seated and facing away from you, move the watch toward the child's ear until ticking is heard; note the distance from watch to ear.

Then put the watch close to the ear where the child reports hearing it and move it away to the point where it becomes inaudible. Note the distance. Repeat for the other ear. Compare distances with someone who has not experienced ear troubles — another child, perhaps, or your spouse. If the distances are substantially lower for the child, tell your doctor, who may order more sophisticated tests by a hearing specialist.

EAR ALLERGIES

Middle ear infections, while they can be caused by allergies, are not allergies as such, and the medications prescribed for treatment of middle ear infections are not aimed at and have no effect on them. However, topical antibiotics put into the ear for treatment of certain local infections — swimmer's itch in particular — can cause a contact allergy, either from the antibiotic or the paste that serves as its vehicle. Your child may be given a topical antibiotic for a superficial ear infection; the ear seems to get better. Then, the skin in the ear canal gets red and the infection seems to grow much worse. Actually, the ear infection is not involved; but an allergic reaction to the antibiotic or its base has set in. If this should happen, discontinue the medication at once and check with your doctor.

TRAVELING WITH AN EARACHE

The eustachian tube is very important in exchanging air between the nose and the ear. If the middle ear begins to become clogged, a fair amount of pain can result. In fact, keeping the eustachian tube open is extremely important. Generally, every time you yawn, chew, or swallow, the tubes open and air is allowed to go through the middle ear. Virtually anyone who has been in an airplane has experienced the popping sensation that occurs as the plane descends to lower altitudes. This is due to the exchange of air between the outside and inside of the ear. In some people with clogged eustachian tubes, especially children, this exchange of air may not occur and intense pain results. The pain can be associated with a temporary loss of hearing and ear infections. Thus, if your child is going to ride in an airplane or travel to the mountains, make sure the ears are clear. If your child is susceptible to ear infections, it would not hurt to administer an over-the-counter antihistamine decongestant before the trip, if your child is old enough to be treated with such a medicine. In fact, one of the very few indications for use of an intranasal decongestant, like Sudafed, is prior to a trip. This treatment, while it is only temporary, may also help open the ear canal.

> Every time Nikki and her family traveled from her home in California's Central Valley to the family summer home in the High Sierras, her daughter developed a severe earache that kept her uncomfortable for several days. It always ruined the family vacation. Finally, after many such episodes, Nikki made the connection between her daughter's ears and high altitude. She saw her doctor, who found that Nikki's daughter had a chronic accumulation of fluid in her middle ear. Nikki was totally unaware that her daughter had been having this problem. Her daughter was treated with antibiotics and antihistamine decongestants and the condition cleared up very rapidly. Afterward, until her daughter reached age eight, Nikki routinely gave her some Actifed before they went up to the mountains. She quickly found that it was only the change in altitude, rather than the altitude itself, that was the problem.

TONSILLECTOMIES AND ADENOIDECTOMIES

Adenoids and tonsils are soft-tissue lymph nodes in the nasal airways. In some children, when enlarged, these structures can cause significant obstruction of the airway and/or constriction of the eustachian tube. When it appears clear beyond doubt that they are implicated in respiratory problems or recurrent ear infections, their surgical removal may be advisable. However, the old practice of routinely taking out tonsils and adenoids has been abandoned as useless if not actually harmful. For some children — those with a cleft palate or who have other speaking problems or handicaps — tonsillectomies or adenoidectomies may seriously impair speech and should be avoided if at all possible.

17.

Allergic and Irritant Contact Dermatitis

Allergic contact dermatitis is an inflammation of the skin characterized by redness and the formation of vesicles; vesicles are similar to blisters. Allergic contact dermatitis occurs after exposure to a wide variety of substances — many of which are also capable of causing *nonallergic* irritation. This *irritant* reaction appears following injury to cells as a result of direct contact with the offending substance; the *allergic* response develops after repeated contacts with a sensitizer, which eventually provokes an immune inflammatory side reaction in the body. In practice it is often difficult to distinguish allergic from irritant contact dermatitis. Table 21 lists ways in which they differ.

Allergic contact dermatitis is much *less* common than the irritant reaction. For example, a substantial proportion of all individuals will display a nonspecific irritating rash when exposed to poison oak, ivy, or sumac, the most common sensitizers; a small number of these individuals will develop allergies to these plants, and they will do so only after a period of seeming immunity — a period, unhappily, during which the allergic reaction is being established.

INCIDENCE

Almost any substance can cause a skin rash in a susceptible person, and almost everyone, at some time or another, touches something that does provoke a reaction. Nobody knows the exact number of individuals suffering from allergic contact dermatitis. We do know that with the

TABLE 21
Symptoms of Two Types of Contact Dermatitis

	TIME TO ONSET AFTER EXPOSURE	*TYPE OF REACTION*	*EXTENT OR DISTRIBUTION*
Irritant contact dermatitis	Rapid — usually within a few hours	Red, scaling, and with blisters; painful	Confined to area of exposure
Allergic contact dermatitits	Slowly — from one day to as long as a week	Red with small pimples; itchy	May spread widely

growing intrusion of chemicals into all aspects of contemporary life the complaint will become more prevalent.

USUAL AGE OF ONSET

Rashes resulting from contact with irritants can occur at any age. Children are especially susceptible to certain irritants — notably feces and urine in diapers and certain chemicals commonly found in and around the house — and they may show symptoms as early as the first few weeks or even days of life. Because allergic reactions usually develop only after repeated exposure over a period of time, dermatitis in infants or very young children is likely to be the irritant type.

SYMPTOMS

Acute contact dermatitis is characterized by itching (often so severe as to be almost unbearable), reddening of the skin, and the eruption of patches of blisters where the irritant has touched the skin. The itching may be accompanied by scaling and crusting if the dermatitis persists or becomes chronic; the skin often thickens and becomes leathery and striated in the affected areas.

CAUSES

If your child contracts contact dermatitis, the chances are fairly good that one of the following agents is responsible:

Body wastes: Urine, feces
Plants: Poison oak, ivy, sumac

Household chemicals: Detergents, polishes, waxes, insecticides, disinfectants

Drugs and medications: Skin medications for cuts, scratches, insect bites, sunburn; topical antihistamines; drugs with names ending in "caine" like *benzocaine*; topical antibiotics, especially penicillin, neomycin

Cosmetics: Toilet soaps, perfumed oils and lotions, lipstick, nail polish, hair dyes

Clothing and footwear: Wool; chemicals applied to garments to retard flame or for sizing; chemicals used in processing or curing leather or rubber footwear

The list above is not meant to be complete; it simply identifies some of the more common causes of contact dermatitis.

FIRST AID AND HOME TREATMENT OF CONTACT DERMATITIS

Effective treatment of your child's contact dermatitis depends on your carrying out two steps successfully. They are

1. Identifying and then avoiding the cause of the reaction
2. Looking after the sores or lesions appropriately

The cause of the reaction can usually be inferred by carefully reviewing the activities or experiences that your child has had recently — especially new or different ones — and trying to link them to the place or places on the body where the lesions have appeared. Figure 6 indicates the places on your child's body where various forms of contact dermatitis are likely to turn up initially. Table 22 lists the most common allergic skin disorders, their causes, and how to treat them.

LONG-TERM TREATMENT

If you pin down the cause of your child's dermatitis accurately, prevent further contact with it, *and* follow the appropriate treatment spelled out in Table 22 faithfully, the problem should be resolved. However, you should see your doctor if

- infection is present;
- the rash, after a few day's treatment, fails to improve or gets worse; or
- you cannot establish the cause. (When the dermatitis is caused by medications or chemicals, the offending agent may be obscure and

FIGURE 6
Common Sites of Contact Dermatitis

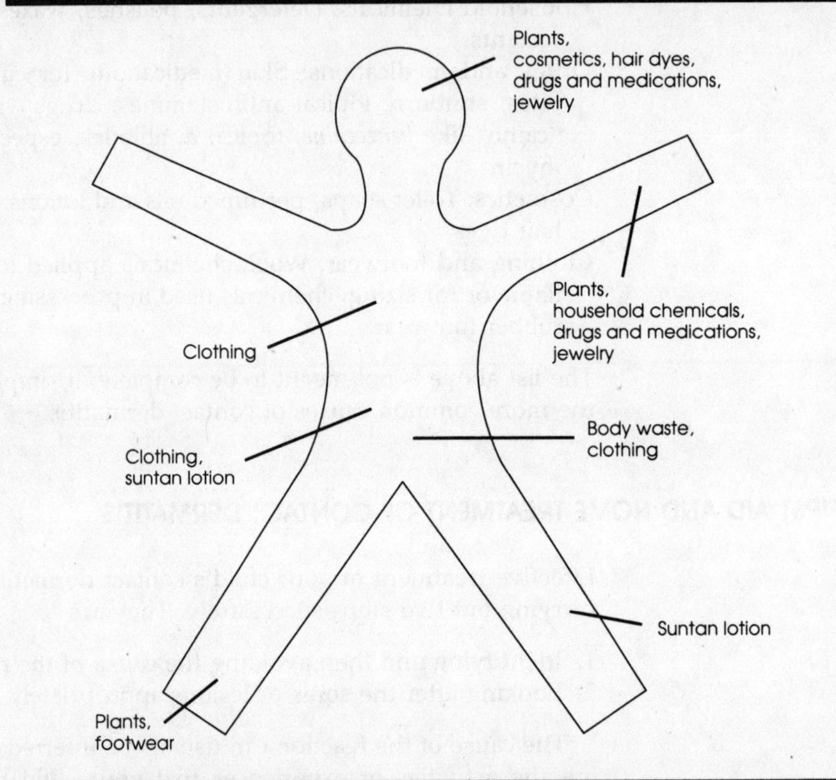

difficult to identify; in these cases accurate diagnosis calls for a patch test which your doctor will have to carry out.)

SPECIAL HINTS

If the cause is correctly identified and the proper treatment is followed, symptoms should clear within a week or two and should not return unless avoidance procedures break down. Normally, contact dermatitis, if treated promptly and effectively, will not cause any permanent damage or disfigurement.

TABLE 22
First Aid and Home Treatment for Common Allergic Skin Disorders

COMPLAINT AND SYMPTOMS	*COMMON CAUSES*	*TREATMENT*
Plant dermatitis (red rash and small blisters; severe itching)	Contact with poison ivy, oak, sumac	1. Learn to identify the plants accurately to avoid them. 2. Avoid contact with pets (dogs especially) that roam in areas where the plants grow. 3. If exposed, flush the site of contact immediately with cold water. 4. If a reaction occurs, apply steroid creams or ointments such as Cortaid. 5. If symptoms are severe and widespread, see a physician for prescription of oral steroid.
Diaper dermatitis (hives and blisterlike pimples in the area covered by the diaper; body folds or creases often less involved)	Overlong contact with feces or urine; soap or detergents remaining in diapers	1. Change diapers frequently. 2. Wash diapers carefully and rinse thoroughly. 3. Clean skin with mild soap and water. Rinse well. If irritation is severe, substitute olive oil or mineral oil for soap. 4. DO NOT use plastic diaper covers. (Plastic-coated disposable diapers, which keep urine away from the skin, are acceptable.) 5. Apply zinc oxide ointment to affected area. 6. If above steps prove ineffectual, consult a physician.
Foot dermatitis (red, thickened, scaly, itchy sores)	Chemicals or other substances used in manufacture of shoes (patch test required for accurate diagnosis)	1. Wear cotton or other nonreactive socks. 2. If necessary, purchase made-to-order, allergy-free footwear. 3. Apply steroid ointment several times daily. Bandage with airtight dressing at night.
Clothing dermatitis (red rash and blisterlike pimples where clothing is in contact with skin)	Wool clothing, overly tight clothing; soaps or detergents remaining in garments; flame-retardant sleepwear	1. Avoid wearing offending fabric. 2. Rinse clothes carefully after washing. 3. If necessary, apply salves or steroid creams or ointments.
Soap and detergent dermatitis (rashing and scaling of skin)	Too frequent or too prolonged bathing; excessive use of bubble bath	1. Bathe less often. 2. Eliminate bubble bath. 3. Use salves or emollients to counteract skin dryness.
Cosmetic and medication dermatitis (rashing, eruption, scaling of skin)	Lipsticks, powders, nail polish, hair dye; names or products or substances ending in "caine" (surfocaine, benzocaine); anti-itch, sunburn, and poison oak remedies; antihistamine and antibiotic ointments and their preservatives (patch test frequently necessary because of number of possible offenders)	1. Avoid use or contact with substance reponsible. 2. Apply steroid salves or ointments.

18.

Headache

INCIDENCE

Headaches are relatively uncommon in childhood. When they do occur, they should be taken seriously because they are often associated with special circumstances that have significant health implications, particularly for allergic children.

USUAL AGE OF ONSET

Headaches can occur at any age. Because their most frequent cause is stress growing out of everyday life, they are much more prevalent in adults.

SYMPTOMS

Children's headaches can be identified roughly according to their perceived location and the nature of the pain itself (Figure 7).

When a child complains that his or her head hurts:

First, determine, if you can, whether the headache is the result of a blow or injury. ("Tell me what happened.") If a trauma is responsible

FIGURE 7 Type of Pain, Usual Location, and Common Causes of Chronic Headache

	USUAL LOCATION			
TYPE OF PAIN	*BOTH SIDES OF HEAD*	*ONE SIDE OF HEAD*	*BEHIND THE EYE*	*ABOVE OR BELOW EYE*
Steady ache	Stress or tension			
Intense, throbbing		Migraine*		
Piercing, burning			Vascular	
Pressurelike				Sinus
CAUSES	Stress; emotional problems; jaw clenching; tooth grinding	Spasms or inflammation of blood vessels; stress	Dietary factors; see Table 23	Sinus infection; congestion of sinuses due to allergy

*Migraine, an extremely complicated condition, has special characteristics. Most migraine sufferers, even before the pain starts, know that it is coming. These preliminary warning symptoms (called the "aura") can include feelings of weakness, lightheadedness, severe nausea, sweatiness or clamminess, dizziness, tremor, extreme sensitivity to sound and light, cold hands and feet. A child with what appears to be migraine should see a neurologist for a firm diagnosis and to have appropriate treatment prescribed.

and it appears serious or if the pain persists for more than a short period of time, call or see your doctor.

Second, have the child indicate the location of the pain ("Where does it hurt?") and its nature. ("Does it hurt all the time?" "Does it come and go?")

These steps are important in identifying the likely cause and deciding what to do about treatment.

CAUSES

In children, the major cause of headache is *fever* — especially a temperature over 103°F (40°C). The fever may be accompanied by nausea and vomiting. Note that fever is a sign or symptom, not a disease in itself. See Chapter 19 for more about fever.

Jay came home from school feeling a bit tired. His baby-sitter was a little surprised that Jay went to the couch and quickly fell asleep. Usually the first thing he did was to turn on the television and watch cartoons. She decided to wake him up after about an hour and ask if he was ill. When aroused he said that he had a very bad headache. He looked flushed and she took his temperature and found it to be 103°F. Jay did not realize he had a fever but, shortly after the baby-sitter took his temperature, he began to vomit. She gave him some Tylenol; his temperature dropped within an hour, and his headache disappeared.

TABLE 23
Foods Containing Vasoactive Amines

1. Chocolate, cocoa, fava beans
2. All ripened cheeses
3. Avocados
4. Bananas
5. Canned figs
6. Fermented sausage (i.e., bologna, salami, pepperoni, aged beef, hot dogs)
7. Red wine, sherry
8. Beer
9. Chicken livers
10. Pickled herring
11. Anchovies
12. Dried fish
13. Yeast extracts (breads and candy)

Headaches may also result from *foods* or other substances that contain chemicals called vasoactive amines. Vasoactive amines cause the blood vessels in the brain to constrict and dilate, and this process produces vascular headache. Table 23 lists foods containing headache-causing vasoactive amines.

In addition, some children may be made violently ill by certain foods that induce nausea, vomiting, or severe diarrhea. This acute *physiological stress* can also cause constriction and dilation of blood vessels and a headache.

A few children will show the acute pain and other symptoms associated with *migraine* headaches. Migraine is also vascular; it runs in families; and it is not the result of allergies. For these reasons, if you suspect that your child has migraine, arrange for a consultation with a neurologist as soon as possible.

Elizabeth has had headaches since she was four years of age. She knows exactly when they will begin. About an hour before the headache she begins to develop a sense of flushing throughout her body. Then, within minutes, ordinary light seems to hurt her eyes. (This pain from light is called photophobia.) Within 15 minutes thereafter, the headache begins. It is an incredibly pounding headache that makes her weak all over, unable to do anything more than lie down in bed. It usually lasts between 4 and 12 hours and only gets better when she takes the special migraine medicine her neurologist prescribed.

Psychological stress — extreme anxiety, tension, conflict — can also produce headache, although these so-called tension headaches are extremely uncommon in children.

Malcolm is considered a brilliant student; he has made virtually straight A's all of his life. He is anxiously awaiting taking his college entrance exams and has been studying very hard for them. It is not uncommon for Malcolm to get headaches. Most often the headaches develop from lack of sleep. Recently, the headaches have been coming on virtually every morning before he goes to school. His mother thinks he is not eating enough and has been trying to feed him more. The result is that he is now becoming obese. Malcolm has confided to his friends that his parents have an obsession about his making high grades and he is afraid that he will fail.

Withdrawal from *caffeine* or caffeine-like substances also causes dilation of blood vessels and a sharp, throbbing headache. While not often encountered in children, it sometimes occurs a few hours after the child has consumed significant amounts of caffeine, especially in soft drinks like cola. It is also seen fairly often in asthmatic children who are taking theophylline, an asthma medication, to control their wheezing.

Hard *physical exertion* — running, jumping, bouts of sneezing, coughing, etc. — is occasionally associated with the sudden onset of, usually short-lived, headaches. And ingesting very cold food or drink (ice cream; chilled soda) can cause a transient headache around the temples.

FIRST AID AND HOME TREATMENT OF HEADACHES

Figure 8 traces the steps to follow in treating your child's headache.

SPECIAL HINTS OR WARNINGS

Aspirin: When a headache hits, most older people immediately think of taking an aspirin. For a child — or for an allergic person of any age — this can be dangerous. *Never, for any reason, administer aspirin to a child.* Use acetaminophin (Tylenol, Datril, Anacin 3, or a generic brand) instead. There are two reasons for this stern advice:

1. Aspirin is associated with Reye's syndrome, an almost always fatal disease in children. It often develops after the use of aspirin to control fever brought on by flu or chicken pox.
2. Aspirin can have severe effects on people with allergies. It can trigger asthma or make it worse, sometimes causing status asthmaticus and hospitalization.

Carl developed asthma following an upper respiratory infection at age three. For the next several years, his asthma always got worse whenever he got a cold. The cold would start in his nose and then move down in his chest. He saw a variety of doctors for this, but no one seemed to help him as much as his family would have liked. He took a whole variety of asthma medications for it, seemingly doing everything he was supposed to. Finally, his pediatrician asked his mom whether Carl ever gets aspirin for fever. She said no,

FIGURE 8
First Aid and Treatment for Headaches

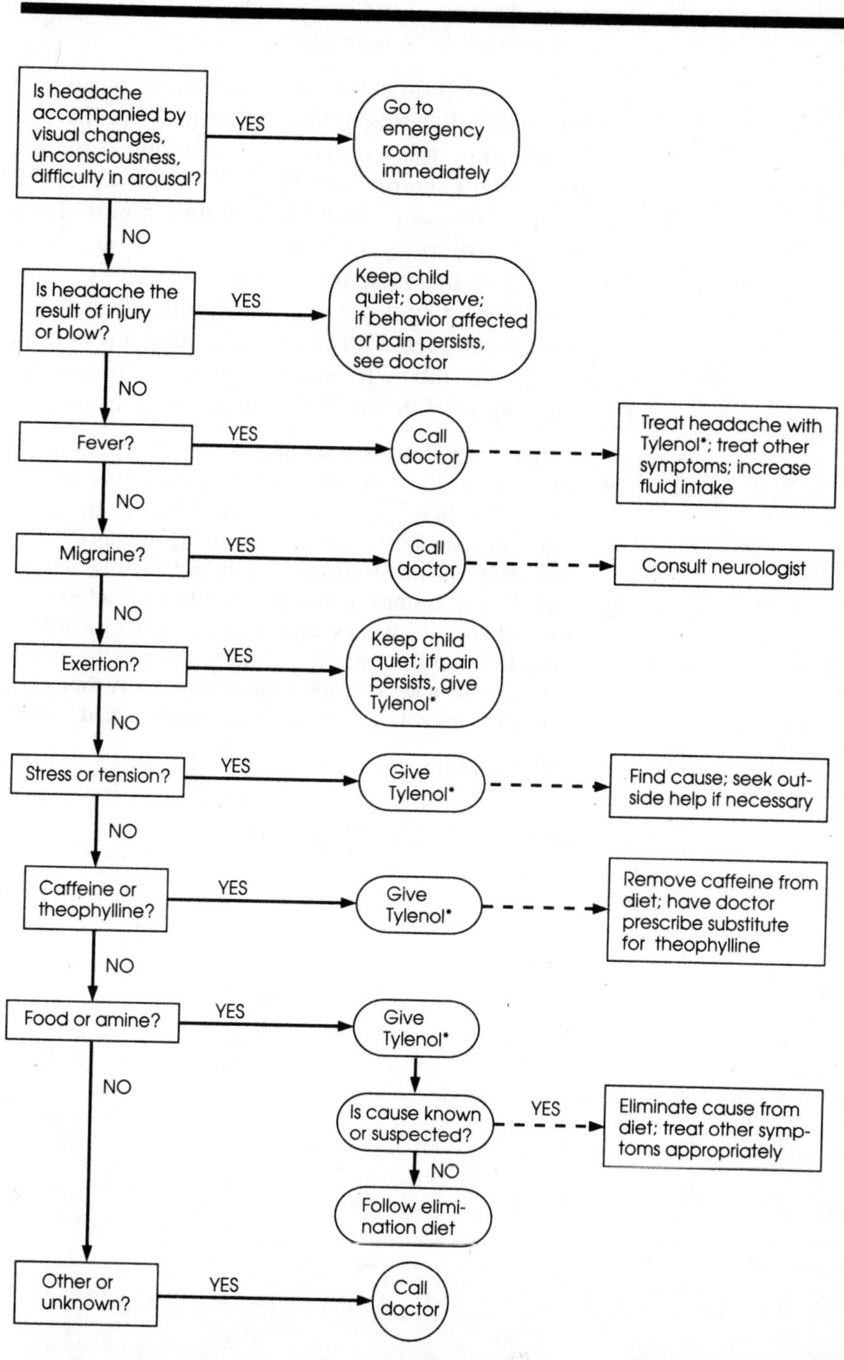

*See text for explanation of Tylenol (acetaminophin) recommendation.

absolutely not. She had been told many times that children with asthma should not be given aspirin. She said she only uses Anacin. *"Anacin!"* the doctor cried. "Anacin contains aspirin!"

In fact, aspirin is found in over 100 medications for colds and congestion, some sleeping pills, and other over-the-counter products. Table 24 lists the kinds of medicine, including some that are used for colds, that contain aspirin. AVOID THESE SCRUPULOUSLY!

"Food" headaches: Don't fall for the claim that headaches are the result of some complex, rare, mysterious reaction to foods. Headache can result from the presence of certain vasoactive amines in the foods named in Table 23. Children who develop headaches without fever should be asked exactly what they have eaten that day and their inventory checked against the table. If matches occur, eliminate the suspected offender and keep track to see if the headache goes away.

Sherry occasionally gets headaches, which always seem to occur about an hour or two after eating cheese. Because her mom is convinced that this is from an allergy to foods, she took Sherry to the doctor to discuss it. Her doctor knows that fresh cheese is rich in vasoactive amines and that Sherry probably has a headache secondary to this; she is just more sensitive to vasoactive amines than other people. He had Sherry write down everything she ate for two weeks, and he also had her record the times of the day when she developed a headache. Sherry realized even before she went back to her doctor that she developed a headache every time she ate fresh cheese. Sherry hated to give it up, but she was certainly glad to get rid of those headaches.

Fortunately, most of us never develop a vasoactive amine headache. For the minority who do, however, missing the diagnosis of the trigger may forbode a life of suffering.

TABLE 24
Common Medicines That Contain Aspirin

- A.P.C.
- Acedyne Wafer
- Aluprin
- Aminodyne Compound
- Anacin
- Analgesic Compound
- Analgestine Forte
- Analgets Water
- Anaphen
- Andquan
- Anexsia-D
- Anodynos-DHC
- Antrin
- Apac
- Apacomp
- Aphonals
- Arthritis Pain Formula
- As-Ca-Phen
- Ascriptin
- Aspergum
- Asphac-G
- Aspir-10
- Aspirbar
- Aspirin
- Aspirin, buffered
- Atokas
- Axotal
- B-A
- Bayer Aspirin
- Bayer Children's Chewable Aspirin
- Bayer Timed-Release Aspirin
- Bexophene
- Buff-A
- Buffadyne-Lemmon
- Bufferin
- Buffex
- Buffinol
- Butalbital Compound
- Butalbital with A.P.C.
- Cafacetin
- Capron
- Carbrogesic
- Christodyne DHC
- Cirin
- Citroval
- Codasa 30mg
- Cold tablets
- Coralsone
- Coricidin
- Dasikon
- Dasin
- Docaphen
- Dolene Compound-65
- Dolor Plus
- Dovacet
- Doverin
- Dovosal
- Drinophen
- Dristan
- Duradyne
- Duragesic
- Dynosal
- Ecotrin
- Emagrin Forte
- Empirin Analgesic
- Emprazil
- Equagesic
- Esemgesic
- Ex Apap
- Excedrin
- Febro-Bar
- Fidgesic
- Fiorinal
- Fizrin
- Gelcoid
- ICN 65 Compound
- Idenal
- I-PAC
- Isobutal
- Isollyl
- Lanabac
- Lanorinal
- Liqualgine
- Marflex Plus
- Margesic Compound No. 65
- Marnal
- Measurin
- Mepro Compound
- Meprogesic
- Methocarbamol with Aspirin
- Micrainin
- Midol
- Momentum
- Nilain
- Norgesic
- Orphenadrine
- P-A-C Compound
- Pain Reliever-E
- Phencoid
- Phenergan Compound
- Phenetron Compound
- Pirseal
- Poxy Compound-65
- Presalin
- Progesic Compound-65
- Propoxyphene Compound
- Proxene Compound
- Pyrroxate
- Quiet World
- Repro Compound-65
- Rhinate
- Rhinex
- Rid-A-Col
- Robaxisal
- Ru-Lor
- Salagen
- Saleto
- Sal-Fayne
- Salocol
- Salphenine
- Sine-Aid Sinus Headache Tablets
- Sine-Off
- SK-65 Compound
- Stanback Analgesic
- Steradrin
- St. Joseph Aspirin
- St. Joseph Aspirin for Children
- Supac
- Synalgos
- Synalgos-DC
- Talwin Compound
- Ten-Shun
- Trigesic
- Valacet
- Valdeine
- Valesin
- Valobar
- Valophen
- Vanquish
- Vasogesic
- Viromed
- Zactirin

19.

Fever

INCIDENCE

Children of any age can, and most at some point do, develop fever. It can appear quickly and, in infants and children, often rises to alarmingly high levels, although children tolerate temperature extremes more readily than adolescents or adults.

SYMPTOMS

A fever is simply an above-normal body temperature. A normal temperature (taken orally) is defined as 98.6°F or 36.9°C. In practice, the healthy individual's temperature will show slight variations from the normal from one day to another and according to the time of day and the type of activity being pursued. Some individuals may have a personal "normal" temperature that is slightly higher or lower than the average 98.6°F.

CAUSES

Fever is a symptom provoked by any of literally hundreds of causes. Infections, colds in particular, are the most common causes of fever. A

TABLE 25
How to Take a Temperature

When using a mercury thermometer:

1. Store the thermometer in its case. (Left loose on the shelf they invariably fall and break; a broken thermometer, even if the mercury column is unaffected, is dangerous.)
2. Before use, dip thermometer in ethyl alcohol to guard against reinfection from prior illnesses.
3. Shake thermometer to drive mercury to base of shaft, near bulb. Check to see that it is down.
4. Insert thermometer. (Temperature may be taken rectally — if proper type of thermometer is used; usually preferable in infants or children 4–6 years old.) In case of rectal administration, lubricate with petroleum jelly; do not force; keep child under close surveillance at all times. In oral administration, place bulb under tongue; keep mouth closed, lips encircling thermometer; caution child *against* biting or moving thermometer.
5. Leave thermometer in place for *at least* 3 minutes.
6. Remove thermometer. Read result. Write down date, time, reading. (This information may be useful for your doctor.)
7. Clean thermometer with cotton, dip in alcohol, shake down, return to case.

Note: When using an electronic or digital thermometer, step 3 is not necessary. In steps 2 and 7, swab with alcohol-soaked cotton before and after use.

fever is an indication that something is wrong. It should *not* be left unattended or trifled with.

Allergies *do not* induce fever. "Hay *fever*" — the popular term for allergic rhinitis — has no effect on body temperature. Like so many other terms in medicine, "hay fever" continues to be widely used, although it is incorrect and misleading.

Even though fever is not the result of allergies, children with allergies may be severely affected by fever because fever accelerates the metabolic rate. Heartbeat and respiratory rate speed up, and these developments can trigger or intensify some allergic conditions — eczema and asthma in particular. Because of this, it is extremely important with allergic children to determine the presence of even a slight fever and to return the body temperature to normal during infections, colds especially.

FIRST AID AND HOME TREATMENT OF FEVER

Treatment of fever has several steps:

1. *Measure the temperature accurately* and record the value, time, and date. See Table 25 for procedures to follow in taking a temperature correctly.
2. *Determine the cause of the fever. Never treat a fever until you are sure what you are treating!* If the condition responsible is not immediately apparent and unmistakable, see the doctor. The reasons for this caution are that the presence of the fever often helps the doctor to diagnose

TABLE 26
Dose of Acetaminophen to Be Administered in Fever

AGE IN YEARS	DOSE*
Less than 2	50mg
2–6	70mg
6–12	150mg
Over 12	375mg

*Can be repeated in 20–30 minutes if no response. Read directions and bottle labels carefully for specific doses.

what is happening. Treating it beforehand may temporarily make the child feel better, but the underlying cause will smolder and get worse. (A child with acute abdominal pain and fever, for instance, can feel better with Tylenol, but if the cause of the fever is appendicitis, appropriate treatment may be delayed, with potentially grave consequences.)

3. *Treat the fever*. Treatment of fever in children consists of *administering acetaminophen* and applying other measures like sponge baths that will lower the surface temperature of the body. The appropriate dosage of acetaminophen is determined by age. Table 26 gives dosages according to age.
4. *Do not treat fever in children with aspirin in any form*. As noted in the preceding chapter, treating fevers with aspirin has been linked with Reye's syndrome, an often fatal disease in children. Aspirin also triggers or intensifies certain allergic reactions, especially asthma, and should not be used by a child or adult who has them. It can also cause bleeding and gastric ulcers.

June has had recurrent colds and infections throughout her childhood. She does not have allergies. Her mother, a nurse, remembers the old days when aspirin was used routinely in hospital patients for fever. She knows not to administer aspirin when the conditions might turn into Reye's syndrome, but no one ever told her that aspirin can induce ulcers. June has been under a fair amount of stress; she has been absent so much during the school year that her work is suffering. She has a temperature of 101°F and her mother has been giving her two aspirin every four to six hours during the daytime. June has been complaining that her stomach has been bothering her and her stools have been turning black and tarry. Her mother thought it might be from the multiple vitamins containing iron. At two o'clock in the morning, June woke up, felt extremely sick, and began to vomit blood. She was rushed to the hospital and diagnosed as having an aspirin-induced ulcer.

5. *Increase fluid intake*. More fluid is needed during a fever.

COMPLICATIONS

Fever, as mentioned above, *can provoke or intensify eczema and asthma.* Monitor the temperature of your asthma- or eczema-prone child regularly and treat even a slight fever promptly. (Eczema symptoms get worse with fever; fever also speeds up breathing, which can lead to hyperventilation and asthmatic wheezing.)

Febrile seizures — seizures that resemble acute epilepsy — sometimes happen in children with high fevers. Children subject to this frightening condition should be watched closely and vigorously treated at the first sign of temperature elevation. This aggressive, preventive posture will usually ward off seizures.

20.

Coughs and Colds

INCIDENCE

Coughing is one of the most frequent problems in children. Most children will have several colds or coughs per year; pharmacy shelves are loaded with over-the-counter cough remedies, many of them aimed at children.

USUAL AGE OF ONSET

Children can turn up with a cough at any age; for allergic children and their parents, colds and coughs take on special significance and need to be watched closely and treated aggressively. The cold/cough–allergy connection is twofold: colds or other respiratory infections are the most common trigger of asthma in children, and a cough is sometimes the only sign of the presence of asthma.

SYMPTOMS

Coughs can take any of several forms and show up at particular times. A cough can be *dry* or *wet*. (A wet cough is one that sounds like it is bringing up phlegm or mucus.) It can be a hoarse *croupy* cough accompanied by noisy, raspy breathing in infants and young children; it can be *around-the-clock* or only at night *(nocturnal)*; or it can be the deep, wracking and unique sound of *whooping cough*, a dangerous but fortunately uncommon childhood disease.

CAUSES

The cough, much like fever or headache, is actually a sign that something is wrong. It may be a reaction to a trivial, everyday infection like a cold or flu, or it may be caused by a serious underlying disease like bronchitis, pneumonia, or whooping cough (*pertussis*), which is brought on through infection by the *Bordetella pertussis* bacterium. Whooping cough has special implications for allergic children and these are discussed under the "Complications" heading later in this chapter.

A chronic cough can also be the result of a foreign object caught in the lung passages — peanuts, M&M's, other food particles, pencil erasers, paper clips, pieces of toys, and so on.

FIRST AID AND HOME TREATMENT OF COUGHS AND COLDS

When Paula picks up her four-year-old daughter Mary from preschool on Wednesday she notices that the child is a bit flushed and somewhat cross. When they get home Paula takes the child's temperature and finds it to be 100.5°F. Mary also begins complaining that her throat hurts. Paula, who knows that many of the children in Mary's room have been troubled by these same symptoms, immediately increases Mary's fluid intake and treats the fever with acetaminophen. Next morning the symptoms have grown more pronounced; while the fever has dropped a bit, Mary now has a cough and a runny nose. Paula keeps her out of school that day, has her stay inside, continues treating the fever, keeps the level of fluid consumption high, and tries to keep her amused without too much success; Mary would rather be at school with her friends. During the day the cough becomes more pronounced and productive — Mary starts bringing up phlegm — so Paula is fairly confident that this is a simple cold. She keeps Mary out of school over the weekend, and by Monday the symptoms are mainly gone and Mary is able to return to school without being actively infectious.

A cough in a child almost always is self-limiting and moderates and goes away by itself after a brief period of time. Steps in the home treatment of a cough are given in Figure 9. Other methods of treatment involve humidifiers and over-the-counter cold and cough medications.

FIGURE 9
First Aid and Home Treatment for Coughs and Colds

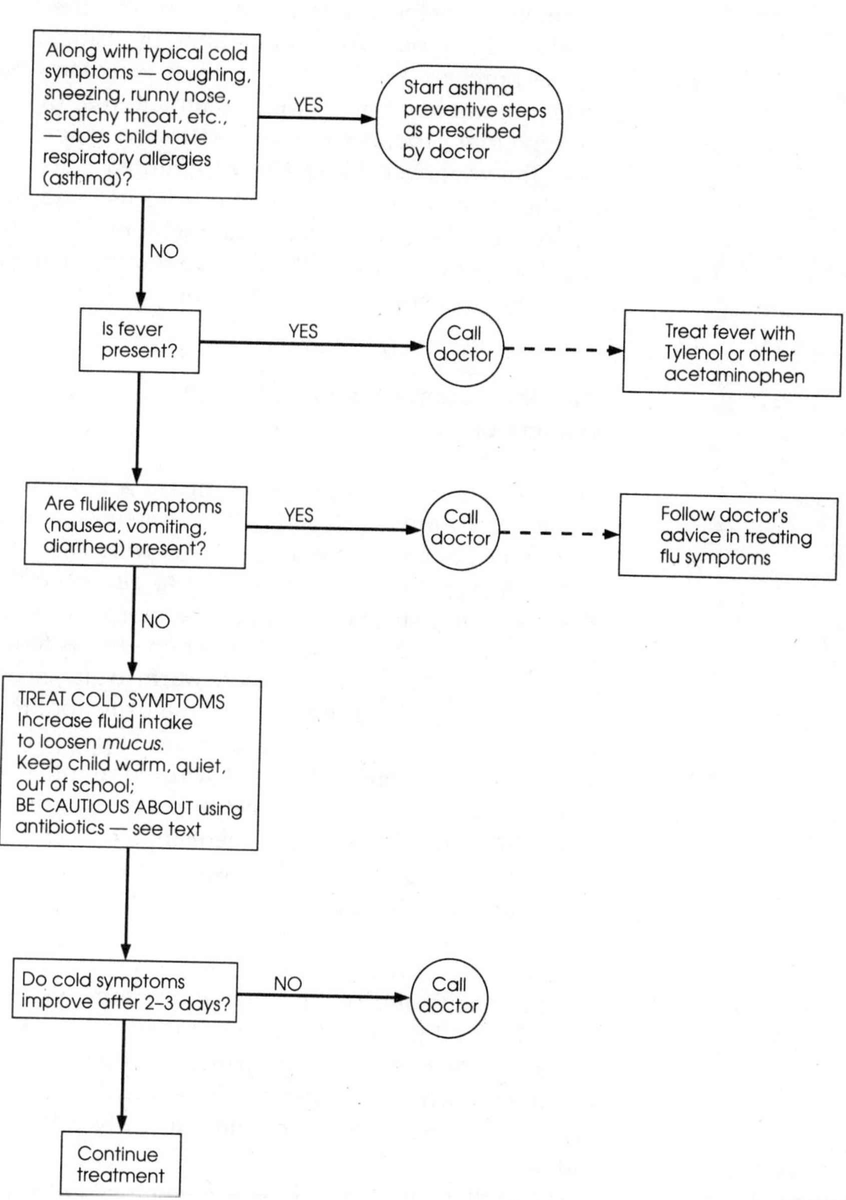

Humidifiers

It sometimes helps, especially in croupy coughs, to increase the humidity of the bedroom. This can be done by using a vaporizer. Vaporizers can be purchased inexpensively from your local pharmacy. To reduce danger of fire and burns, we recommend that the vaporizer you use be the type that produces room-temperature vapor. It is also important to clean the vaporizer *thoroughly* with diluted vinegar (both the container *and* the vaporizing mechanism) during use and before storing it; otherwise it can become contaminated with mold or other allergens, which in subsequent use enter the air to aggravate coughs and trigger other symptoms in asthmatics and hay fever sufferers.

Over-the-Counter Cold and Cough Medications

Over-the-counter medications come in a bewildering variety of brand names and forms — liquids, pills, capsules, lozenges. There are two main types of cough medication — *suppressants* and *expectorants*.

Cough suppressants are supposed to eliminate the cough. To do this they rely on a substance called dexomorphan, but its concentration in children's over-the-counter cough remedies is too small to be effective. Having the youngster sip clear, warm fruit juices or a mild herb tea with honey can be as effective as the drugstore remedies.

Cough lozenges or drops that are supposed to ease coughing are little more than candy flavored with eucalyptus or horehound to give it a medicinal taste. You can get the same mouth and throat-moistening effect from fruit Life-Savers. There are effective cough suppressants but they can only be obtained on prescription. These medications are potent, carry heavy side effects, and are not routinely recommended for children.

Cough expectorants are supposed to act to lubricate and help get rid of the mucus and other material accompanying a cold or respiratory infection. While the idea is fine in principle, expectorants are not especially effective. A sharp increase in fluid intake will usually accomplish as much at considerably less cost. By "sharp increase" we mean at least double or triple the normal daily intake of (preferably) warm liquids.

Note that some expectorants contain an antihistamine and may have an alcohol base as well. These formulations can have the effect of causing drowsiness or sleepiness which, in asthmatic children, can impair breathing efficiency and trigger a severe bout of asthma. The antihistamines may also dry out the nose and eustachian tube and bring on earache (otitis media) or severe and stubborn nasal symptoms in susceptible children.

COMPLICATIONS

Whooping cough, once widely prevalent, is a serious, sometimes fatal disease of childhood; mortality rates of as high as 50% have been recorded. Children who contract this disease develop a severe cough often associated with a deep breath or "whoop" just before the cough — hence its name. In instances where it proves fatal, the cough becomes nonstop, preventing the child from taking in any air and, in effect, causing the child to suffocate.

There is a preventive vaccine for whooping cough as well as an effective antibiotic treatment. We believe that every normal child should complete the whooping cough immunization series; however, the whooping cough vaccine carries special, serious implications for allergic children. Our reasons for concern have to do with some unusual properties of the whooping cough vaccine. It has been shown, in animals, to be an *adjuvant,* that is, in addition to conferring immunity to *Bordetella pertussis* it is capable of inducing high levels of IgE. A high level of IgE in humans can make allergies worse.

Because of this adjuvant property, we recommend that children with moderate to severe allergies and a family history of allergies, *as well as* all children with asthma, *not* receive whooping cough vaccine. (See Chapter 24 for recommendations on vaccination.) Other allergic children should *not* be vaccinated when they have a cold or other respiratory infection or at times when pollen counts are high.

We recommend that you talk over this problem, if it applies to your child, with your pediatrician or family practitioner. If the doctor seems unaware of the whooping-cough vaccine–IgE link, have him or her discuss it with an allergist before making a decision.

SPECIAL HINTS

Nocturnal cough, a cough that occurs at night with no other symptoms, may be the first and sometimes the only sign of asthma. You, the parent, may resort to treating this annoying sort of cough with any of hundreds of over-the-counter cough medications — usually with no success. The only effective treatment will be one that addresses the underlying asthma.

For children with a nocturnal, asthma-caused cough we recommend treatment at bedtime with asthma medication as prescribed by your pediatrician or family practitioner. Usually this preventive treatment will make the cough go away. Since the mildest form of asthma is ordinarily implicated in nocturnal cough, it usually vanishes as the child grows older — often by the age of six years or so — and the respiratory airways enlarge.

21.

Other Allergic and Pseudo-Allergic Complaints

Allergy has always been one of the most difficult specialties in medicine. There are a number of reasons for this. First, the antibody IgE, which triggers many of the symptoms of allergy, is present in the blood in such very small quantities that it was not until 1966 that it was even detected and its role in causing allergic symptoms revealed. Second, many physicians and scientists found it inconceivable that the body's immune system might do harm to the body. Indeed, even anaphylaxis — the severe and sometimes fatal reaction susceptible people have to bee stings, certain medications, and so on — was not accepted as a medical condition even though the symptoms had been known for centuries. Only with the work of Bertha Schick in the early part of this century was anaphylaxis defined as a disease entity. Third, too many people — physicians among them — wrongly conclude that any condition that resists diagnosis has to be allergic in origin. As a result, allergy has become a catchall diagnosis for a wide variety of baffling conditions, and a steady parade of men, women, and children complaining of a myriad of vague, mysterious symptoms turn up at the allergist's office. This tendency to turn allergy into the Ellis Island of diseases has been encouraged by a parallel development; with the accelerating degradation and invasion of the environment by substances that do cause symptoms, allergic and hypersensitivity reactions are on the increase.

There are a variety of problems we all encounter in everyday life as we face daily stresses, and the extent of their impact is not clearly known. Perhaps in the twenty-first century we will come to know more about the causes and management of conditions like stress, headaches, depression, agitation, fatigue, hyperactivity, inability to concentrate, and the like. For now, though, these are simply words that strive to describe how one feels — and not at all precisely at that. The sections that follow discuss some of these common syndromes and what we know about them.

ALLERGIC FATIGUE OR ALLERGIC TENSION-FATIGUE SYNDROME

This syndrome was first described nearly 30 years ago as extreme fatigue often associated with agitation or hyperactivity. With some individuals these periods of fatigue and hyperactivity seem to be concurrent; in others, one of the conditions will persist for days or even weeks at a time only to be supplanted by the other. These conditions are often seen in children.

Some attribute these symptoms to food allergy or to environmental chemicals. While this is an attractive hypothesis, there is no evidence that indicates that the syndrome is in fact due to allergies to food or anything else. There are many people, children and adults, who go through or experience recurring bouts of fatigue and hyperactivity. The symptoms often add up to a problem that interferes with school work, job performance, or family life. It is a serious condition that may require medical attention, attention that may in the end fail to pin down a cause. Nonetheless, there is no evidence at all that any allergic disease, allergic phenomenon, or any component of the immune system is involved.

Individuals with this syndrome have been targeted by unscrupulous practitioners (physicians as well as a variety of other specialists, legitimate or self-proclaimed) offering exotic, excessive, and usually ineffectual treatments. Be very careful when seeking treatment for this condition.

DEPRESSION, PSYCHOSIS, AND NEUROTIC BEHAVIOR

There are physicians who describe themselves as clinical ecologists. Their practice is founded on the belief that contact with chemicals, preservatives in food, food itself and its products can significantly affect the nervous system. As we have repeatedly pointed out, what we ingest can affect our behavior. Some foods cause headaches in susceptible persons; specific allergy or sensitivity to certain foods can produce colic, diarrhea, hives, itching, and other allergic reactions. Nonetheless, there is no evidence that food products, chemicals, or preservatives can bring about the psychiatric symptoms — neurosis and depression — that the ecologists say they produce. While we are not beyond being persuaded that such may be the case, we know of no data to support the belief.

We do know that people exposed to certain toxins, the metal lead, for example, have long been known to develop extensive pathology including diseases of the nervous system. However, not only do toxins like lead have specific behavioral effects that have been catalogued, but, most important, their presence can be detected in the body and is reflected in measurable changes in the blood, the bone marrow, and sometimes the kidney. No such observations or measurements have been offered by the clinical ecologists. In the absence of scientific data to support their hypotheses and their therapeutic regimens, we have no enthusiasm for them and recommend that they be avoided.

THE YEAST CONNECTION

Another group of physicians assert that a raft of psychological or physical symptoms are due to the fact that we have become allergic to yeast, or candida. They offer dietary and other treatments, some of them quite bizarre, that are billed as managing the hypothetical generalized invasion of the body by yeast. The alleged yeast connection is based on anecdotal information with very poor documentation. There are no controlled scientific studies to support their musings. Yet, much like the clinical ecologists, the yeast faddists seem to offer an easy out. We are deeply skeptical of this approach; pursuing it will certainly turn out to be expensive, probably ineffectual, and possibly harmful, especially when it denies your child the benefits of a medically sound approach.

ARTHRITIS

There have been scattered medical reports that arthritis is made worse by certain foods, particularly milk. The Arthritis Foundation has conducted numerous studies of the possible relationship of food to arthritis. It is possible that a small number of people with arthritis show sensitivity to specific foods, but the bulk of the evidence indicates that food allergy alone is not a cause of arthritis. This is also true of other diseases as well, including irritable bowel syndrome, Crohn's disease, and systemic lupus erythematosus.

BED-WETTING

There are a number of causes of enuresis, or bed-wetting. Some of them may be serious and organically caused, reflecting problems in the urogenital system. Others are simply a matter of maturity and go away as the child develops. There is no evidence that bed-wetting is related in any way to allergies. There are, however, some allergy medications that increase urine output and make bed-wetting more of a potential problem. One of these is theophylline, a drug commonly used to treat asthma. Theophylline, in addition to dilating the airways and relieving breathing difficulties, stimulates the kidney to make more urine. Since asthmatic children routinely take theophylline at bedtime, it is not unusual for such children to need to urinate during the night. Since children tend to sleep profoundly, the result may be bed-wetting. If this occurs and your child is on theophylline, we think it important for you to discuss the problem with your family doctor or pediatrician and obtain alternative medication.

DEALING WITH PROBLEMS EFFECTIVELY

One of the best resources to have in dealing with obscure or mysterious symptoms in your child is an understanding and painstaking physician. Too many doctors predicate their practices on writing prescriptions and ordering lab tests. The problems enumerated above require a great deal of doctor or nurse attention. They use up large bites of time from busy practices, and the fees generated for such evaluations are usually not as high as those that come in by doing standard procedures and seeing more patients per unit of time. For good physicians who are dedicated to helping their patients, time is not a factor. We have found that one of the most effective ways to deal with problems like these is to help the family understand and to learn to cope with them directly. In so doing it is amazing how many of these problems gradually fade away.

Understanding and a good measure of hope and optimism about these complaints can often be found in patient encounter groups, parent support groups, or an aggressive program of self-education aimed at understanding and learning to manage the symptoms. Unhappily, all too often parents, understandably beleaguered, look for a quick fix, turning to practitioners who offer overnight cures. This tactic may provide some short-run psychological help and make child and parent feel better briefly, sustained by the belief that they have found somebody with a magic cure for their problem. Usually the quick-fixed problem comes back, more stubborn than ever on reappearance. We think parents of children with these chronic, troublesome problems should be especially cautious when it comes to choosing a physician and should read and follow the suggestions in Chapter 22 carefully.

PART FOUR

GETTING THE BEST, MOST EFFECTIVE LONG-TERM CARE FOR YOUR ALLERGIC CHILD

22.

Looking After Your Allergic Child

Although health care delivery systems are undergoing a lot of change, primary responsibility for the care of the allergic child still rests with you, the parent. This is particularly true if you are in a Health Maintenance Organization or rely, as so many do, on an emergency room or clinic. Under these conditions there may be little or no continuity in outside care. Whether or not there is continuity in medical care, you are the very best — perhaps only — person to know what is really happening with your child, and you certainly have the keenest interest and the largest stake in seeing to it that she or he is helped. It is up to you to become educated and involved in your child's care and to find out what the problem is, its causes, its treatment, and, most important, its prevention. The first step in providing sound care is to find the right doctor.

WHAT TO LOOK FOR IN A PHYSICIAN

Virtually every family doctor or pediatrician will faithfully carry out routine aspects of care — weighing children in, inquiring about eating habits and school adjustment, discussing physical and social development, treating the occasional rash or fever, and looking after the immunization series advocated by the American Academy of Pediatrics. Much of this care can also be provided by well-trained family nurse practitioners or physician assistants. The key element in the medical care of the majority of children entails learning to recognize the acutely ill child who requires urgent and aggressive treatment and knowing when and how to use appropriate remedies judiciously.

For children with allergies, the choice of a physician becomes a much different matter. Allergies are likely to persist throughout childhood and well into adolescence, and they sometimes turn out to be a lifelong problem. Children with allergies see their physicians more often, they have more colds and other respiratory infections, and they are quite prone to have multiple allergies, all above and beyond the ordinary problems that other children have. If you have an allergic child it is vital that you become intimately involved in choosing your child's physician and then participating in the ongoing care for the condition. Here are some important matters to consider when choosing a doctor for your allergic child.

1. *Do you feel comfortable with your doctor?*

Is your doctor inclined to be brusque and hurried, or does he or she take time to respond to your questions and concerns fully and understandably? To what extent are you provided with literature on your child's problem? There are excellent booklets available from groups like the American Academy of Allergy and Immunology and the American Allergy Association on allergies and asthma (see Appendix H). Your doctor can easily arrange for and in fact should see to your receiving these informational/instructional materials.

2. *Is the doctor a graduate of an accredited American medical school?*

There are, of course, many outstanding physicians who are graduates of foreign medical schools, but we believe that, in choosing a graduate of an American medical school, you can be sure he or she has met certain minimum criteria of training and competence. In U.S. medical schools standards are strict and reasonably uniform. Your librarian will direct you to a list of accredited medical schools.

3. *Is your doctor well trained and board certified to practice as a family physician, pediatrician, allergist, or other specialist?*

Upon graduation from medical school the new doctor receives a diploma that declares that its recipient can now practice medicine and surgery. But in truth the new graduate cannot practice anything. He or she must first pass rigorous written examinations — state or national boards, depending on the part of the country. In addition, graduating physicians must, at the very least, complete one year of postgraduate training, known as an *internship*. Following successful completion of the internship they are eligible to practice medicine. Once these new young doctors would have gone out into the world as general practitioners. In fact there are very few young general practitioners anymore, because most physicians recognize the need for additional training in specialties such as family practice, internal medicine, pediatrics, and surgery. These programs require from two to five additional years, depending on the specialty. Once this advanced training phase is completed they take another examination, and if they pass they become specialists in the area they chose. Thus, a family practitioner will have on her wall a certificate testifying that she passed her board certification by the American Board of Family Practice. And a pediatrician or internist will display in his office similar testimony from the American Board of Pediatrics or the American Board of Internal Medicine. Some physicians, a minority, elect to train even further in a subspecialty such as allergy and immunology, chest diseases, or one within surgery like orthopedics. Once again stiff exams are required at the close of this phase of training.

What all this means is that a properly qualified allergist, for instance, should have at the very least

- certification of having passed the American Board of Internal Medicine or American Board of Pediatrics requirements, and
- certification of having passed and been certified by the American Board of Allergy and Clinical Immunology.

Ask the doctor or nurse about the doctor's specialty and certification status. Get a definite yes or no answer to your question. Do not accept or be misled by the statement that the doctor is "board eligible" but has not yet taken the exam — *unless* he or she is a new arrival in the community. Such newcomers are entitled to a period of grace before they have to sit for their exam. Also, do not take your allergic child to other specialists, such as an "ear, nose, and throat" doctor. If you want the best, see a board-certified allergist, not a generic substitute.

4. *Do not wait until sickness strikes to choose a doctor; make your choice when your child is well.*

Select a pediatrician, family practitioner, or physician during pregnancy. (Health Maintenance Organizations and company health plans allow for this type of choice.) Talk to family, friends, and co-workers about likely possibilities. Then, ask for an appointment to introduce yourself and to check out the doctor. You will find that all doctors are willing to meet you and discuss their practice and office procedures. This first meeting is a good time to check on training and board certification. It is also a good time to find out about the cost of visits and about attitudes toward treatment. Be sure the physician is concerned about prevention, not just about treating you or your child when sick. He or she should ask you questions about your dietary and health habits. You should be asked about feeding plans or procedures — breast or formula.

If your initial visit is with your newborn, the doctor should inquire about weight, eating behavior, sleep patterns, and so on. It should be absolutely clear to you that the doctor puts the highest priority on preventing rather than treating illness.

5. *Find out about emergency care.*

Does your doctor close up shop at five o'clock? Who covers during off-duty hours? Are you told to go to the local hospital emergency room? Or is your doctor associated with a group of physicians who provide regularly staffed acute care coverage after hours and on weekends? To what extent is telephone consultation permitted and encouraged? Can you call your physician for advice, or do you have to bring your child in? (Many good physicians reserve an hour during the day for telephone calls and consultation with their patients.) In short, is your doctor ready and willing to provide the kind of help you need whenever it is needed? If so, fine; if not, look elsewhere.

6. *Get what you are paying for.*

Any good doctor will allow a minimum of 30 minutes for a first examination. It should include a complete, detailed history that includes a family history, mother's health during pregnancy, childhood illnesses, and school attitudes and performance. There should also be a complete examination — looking in the eyes and ears and listening to the chest. Where skin problems are concerned, the whole body should be looked at, and children must be asked to strip down to their underwear so that no part of the skin goes unobserved. In the case of asthma and hay fever, the detailed examination should include the nose and feeling of pulses, right to the extremities, fingers and toes. Where indicated, it may also include laboratory tests and possibly chest or sinus X rays.

CHOOSING A SUBSPECIALIST

Children who have stubborn and serious allergic problems such as chronic eczema and moderate to severe asthma should be seen by a specialist. Although most primary care physicians like pediatricians and family practitioners are well equipped to take care of mild allergic conditions, we believe that care of chronic conditions requires evaluation and treatment by someone who has specialized training. Consulting a specialist helps to affirm the accuracy of the diagnosis while assuring you that your child is receiving the most up-to-date treatment and that treatment plans will be modified to reflect the development of new therapies or the introduction of new medications.

There are three specialists most often involved in the care of allergic children: allergists, dermatologists, and pediatric chest physicians. Each of these has received the additional training necessary for and should display the board certification covered earlier in this chapter.

Children who have eczema need to see a dermatologist who will usually be someone recommended by your family doctor. However, in choosing a dermatologist, you ought to observe the same procedures that you followed in choosing your doctor to begin with, by inquiring about board certification and so forth. If you do not feel comfortable with the first person you consult, make another choice. Most communities have a number of dermatologists (the Yellow Pages of the telephone directory or the local medical society lists these and other specialists).

Deciding between an allergist and a chest physician is often more difficult. For routine allergies that do not involve asthma, one should generally consult an allergist. An allergist should have board certification and be capable of making the appropriate decisions regarding skin testing, of prescribing appropriate medical therapy, and of addressing the issues of environmental control and preventive measures that are so important to the management of allergies.

As a group, allergists are well trained and their level of proficiency is far better than it was 15 or 20 years ago, before the recent and dramatic advances in the field. Even so, there is a pitfall that some patients may encounter. Some allergists base their fees on the number of skin tests they conduct. As a result, they carry out more allergy tests than is medically necessary or even advisable. You do not want your child to become a veritable pincushion unless extensive testing is clearly indicated. Chapter 2 covers allergic evaluation. Review it if the question of skin testing comes up so that you can be involved in this decision process. Be forewarned if the doctor begins the evaluation by bringing out a tray of skin test materials, even before taking a detailed history and doing a physical examination. These two preliminary steps can often determine the cause of an allergy without your doctor having to resort to skin testing at all.

Severe childhood asthma requiring periodic hospitalization or emergency room care should be treated by a specialist in chest medicine. For one thing, in infancy and early childhood there are some grave causes of asthma that include cystic fibrosis and a rare disease known as gastroesophageal reflux (GER); both of these conditions require skilled, specialized attention. For another, should your child require hospitalization, it is likely that it will be your pediatric chest physician who will care for your child during the acute hospitalization phase.

Unhappily, there is a shortage of trained pediatric chest specialists; many communities have none at all. In that event, a child with chronic asthma may be referred to a specialist in adult chest medicine or to an allergist.

BEING A RESPONSIBLE PARENT

There have been scores of books written about effective parenting, and we have no intention of summarizing them here. We simply want to emphasize that, to care for your allergic child effectively, you need to develop the skill, knowledge, and resolve necessary to make decisions about your child yourself. You have to learn to be a responsible parent and to guide your child to be a responsible patient.

When you bring your child to the doctor, make sure that you tell the doctor everything in all the detail that you can. So that you do not forget, write down details of symptoms — what, when, where, how much — before you show up for the consultation. Be very clear. Doctors often try to relax you by easing you into a gentle and probably irrelevant conversation. Do not let this divert you. You are there because you and your child have a problem. Discuss it!

Once the reason for the visit is established and treatment decided on, there are a number of questions you should have answered. (It helps, in following and evaluating treatment, to write the answers down.)

1. What is the diagnosis?
2. How long will the condition last?
3. What are the drugs that have been prescribed? What are their possible side effects? How long does the doctor think it will take for the drugs to work? How long will my child need to take the drugs? How exactly ought they be administered (how much, when, by what means)?
4. When should I call if treatment does not help?
5. Should I make a follow-up appointment to see the doctor? When?
6. Is the condition serious enough to warrant seeing a specialist or getting a second opinion?
7. Is there anything I should be doing at home to the environment, diet, and so on, to make the symptoms better?
8. How soon before my child can return to school?
9. What should be done about administering medication during the day, at school?

PSYCHOLOGICAL ASPECTS OF CARE FOR ALLERGIC CHILDREN

The popular belief that some forms of allergic disease (asthma and stomach disorders in particular) are psychologically caused is without foundation. Extensive, careful scientific research has been unable to find any causal connection between psychological states and wheezing, for instance. Other equally rigorous studies have failed to demonstrate that psychotherapy in its various forms relieves allergic symptoms.

However, there is a chicken-egg question here; while it is true, for example, that anxiety does not produce the symptoms of asthma or eczema, asthma and eczema can — and often do — provoke psychological reactions that carry physical consequences that can intensify the ongoing allergic reaction. Children with moderate to severe asthma have to fight for every breath. The experience is terrifying; youngsters having a moderate to severe attack frequently wonder if they are going to last through the night. This fear and the associated struggle for breath causes rapid, shallow breathing — hyperventilation — that triggers further spasms in the smooth muscles that surround the respiratory airways and compromises the breathing even more. Thus, fear and hyperventilation combine in a vicious circle.

Children with eczema or other allergic skin complaints experience intense itching. What do you do with an itch? Scratch it. What happens when you scratch an allergic itch? Usually it gets worse. This upward spiral of intense discomfort is frustrating, depressing, and anxiety-producing. These reactions can affect the vascular system, resulting in increased production of perspiration that, in its turn, aggravates the already agonizing itching.

It is also evident that allergies can be associated with conflict in the family or home setting. Some of these conflicts arise out of the resistance of the allergic child to the care regimen being administered by the parents; others are associated with simple disagreements — personality clashes that are brought on or intensified because of a chronic allergic disease. These conflicts can be severe enough to produce the kinds of reactions we have described above. Conflict does not in itself cause allergies, but it can set off physiological reactions that make the condition worse.

Thus, through what can be thought of as a kind of feedback loop, an allergic reaction can provoke psychological reactions that act to intensify the original symptoms. This sort of problem can be managed fairly easily with appropriate medication or by adopting other tactics (e.g., in asthma, diaphragmatic breathing and stress-reducing exercises) that address the primary symptoms. Each of Chapters 10 through 21 contains a section that presents measures that relieve primary allergic symptoms.

SECONDARY PSYCHOLOGICAL EFFECTS ON PARENTS

There is a widely held yet erroneous belief that allergies in children stem from psychological causes rooted in malparenting, and it has caused a lot of unnecessary grief. Parents who believe this myth — and there are millions who still do — experience an enormous amount of self-destructive guilt. They needlessly blame themselves for the troubles their kids are having, and they want but are unable to figure out what they have done wrong so that they can right matters. This parental guilt is probably the most pervasive and severe consequence of allergic disease in children. The obvious antidote is to come to the firm realization that, although they may have passed along genes that made their kids subject to allergies, nothing else they did or did not do caused the symptoms. This is something most parents have difficulty with.

The task of caring for an allergic child also has its psychological fallout. The symptoms themselves can be immensely frightening; watching an asthmatic child fight to breathe, not knowing quite what to do to help, or having done all that one can without apparent effect, is extremely upsetting. The symptoms that affect the respiratory system or the skin almost invariably disturb and disrupt the child's (and parents') sleep patterns, producing stress, frustration, even anger. And the need to be constantly aware of and vigilant about avoiding or controlling triggers calls for not only unceasing alertness but sometimes a heavy addition to the work load at home. This, too, can heighten tension and cause conflict within the family.

Care for an allergic child can disrupt work, recreation, and other family activities; it may even create a situation in which the parents feel that their other nonallergic children are being deprived of their fair share of care and attention. A moderate to severe allergy can so sensitize parents that they become unnecessarily — even dangerously — overprotective of the ailing child.

All of these factors can demoralize parents, heighten conflict within the family, and help set off anxiety or depressive reactions. Allergies, in short, can wreak psychological havoc in the family.

Parents can control damage from psychological fallout by applying a combination of knowledge and ameliorative strategies. Here are things you can do to keep your life on an even keel when faced with the care of an allergic child.

1. Understand at the outset that you and your spouse could not have caused the child's symptoms.
2. Learn as much as you can about the disease — what causes it, and what you and the child can do to avoid it, to recognize its early warning symptoms, and to treat it. (You will need help from your doctor to do this; see also the relevant chapters in Part III of this book.)
3. To the extent possible, share information about the nature and cause of the disease with your child. Whenever feasible, have the child assume at least some level of responsibility for observing avoidance tactics and making treatment decisions.
4. Keep in mind that the child is not to blame for the condition, may be extremely uncomfortable with and frightened by it, and certainly doesn't want it.
5. Distribute the care of the child as equitably as possible. Both parents, where present, should be directly involved in the care of the ailing child, sharing in all its aspects.
6. Try not to become overprotective, in effect, enveloping the child in a cocoon. It will only add to your labors and stretch out your problems.
7. If interpersonal conflict between any combination of allergic child, parents, and other children erupts, move immediately to work through and resolve the problem as harmoniously as possible.
8. Learn how to recognize and cope with your own stress. There are any number of ways to do this, from exercise and physical activity to hobbies, to discussing the situation with another person, to biofeedback, to meditation, to counseling or therapy. Sometimes medication such as tranquilizers can help, but steer clear of alcohol, and beware of becoming chemically dependent.
9. Keep in mind that the symptoms are quite likely to be short-lived, can almost certainly be treated successfully, and probably won't carry any long-term effects.

SECONDARY PSYCHOLOGICAL EFFECTS ON CHILDREN

Children with allergies can experience a variety of secondary psychological reactions that may complicate the original allergic picture. In some instances these psychological reactions, such as anxiety, will carry physiological side effects, such as hyperventilation, that act to worsen the allergic reaction. But there are other possible psychological side reactions as well, such as malingering, reactions to medication, feelings of inadequacy or depression, and a disposition to test the limits insofar as medication or treatment is concerned.

Malingering, that is, using the allergic condition to get out of something unpleasant, is seen fairly often.

> Mrs. B. notes that her son Keith, now 12, complains every Tuesday that he is having an asthma attack. She is suspicious of this because the symptoms are mild and clear up completely by evening. She checks with the school and talks with the principal and with Keith's teachers. The PE instructor mentions the fact that on Tuesdays he brings in a guest teacher who puts the boys and girls through a program of gymnastic exercises that include vaulting, acrobatics, and trampoline work. The instructor goes on to say that Keith obviously dislikes this session and, because he has such difficulty doing some of the stunts, he is teased unmercifully by his classmates. Mrs. B. discusses this problem with Keith, who finally grudgingly admits that his convenient symptoms were largely put on to spare him embarrassment at school.

Where malingering is suspected, try to find out the reason for the behavior and then to do something about its cause. If the reason is not apparent, then it may be that the home situation is simply more congenial than the alternatives and a "time out" from positive reinforcement may correct the matter. This entails withdrawing some of the amenities that make staying at home preferable to carrying out other activities. Confine the child to room and bed, withdraw television, radio, hi-fi, video, or other games, withhold attention, deny access to telephone, and so on — in short, make the child act in a fashion consistent with the claim of illness.

Reactions to medication often take on psychological overtones. Use of antihistamines especially can cause drowsiness and lassitude; other medications can cause your child to be irritable, jittery, even hyperactive.

To deal with these drug-related conditions, first make sure that you know the potential side effects of any medication your allergic child is taking. If one turns up, contact the physician who prescribed the medication at once and ask for further instructions. For most allergic conditions where treatment can produce psychological side reactions there are alternative medications available. These (while they may be more costly or more difficult to administer) will not cause the youngster to go into a daze or become so hyperactive that you cannot deal with the situation.

Feelings of inadequacy or depression can grow out of some severe, chronic, and stubborn allergic conditions — asthma, skin allergies, and hay fever, in particular. Moreover, simply knowing that one must spend an entire lifetime watching out for a trigger like food dye or peanut butter is enough to provoke feelings of depression.

Where such feelings can be traced to the disease itself, you can best help your child by giving her the opportunity and the support she needs to participate in substitute activities that are both satisfying and ego-boosting. For every forbidden pursuit there are literally hundreds of such satisfying alternatives that are both challenging and safe.

Finding acceptable substitutes may take some time and effort on your part, both to narrow down the wide array of possibilities and then to get your youngster started on one or two. But beginning and staying with the ones preferred will prove to your child to be a rewarding activity, better, certainly, than sitting around nursing feelings of inadequacy or depression.

Testing the limits is something individuals with any form of chronic disease are continually tempted to do — just to see if the underlying condition, possibly controlled by medication or otherwise quiescent, has gone away. Nobody wants to be dependent on medication or to have their activities curtailed for any reason.

For those people with allergic diseases, this temptation is particularly strong, because their health is not compromised in any way when the allergic symptoms are controlled or dormant. It's almost as if the disease never happened. So, they say, "I think I've got this thing licked," and, to test the hypothesis, do something that puts them at risk. People have a powerful need to think of themselves as being whole and in control, and so, since most allergies are mild, usually no harm results from this sort of experimentation. But where a serious, chronic condition is being played with in this way, there may be dire consequences. We ardently wish that children with these chronic diseases (and their parents) would trust us on this one. The symptoms may not be around right now, they may not be as bad as they once were, and maybe they aren't giving as much trouble as they used to. Let well enough alone. Don't find out the hard way that the underlying condition is still lurking, waiting to pounce.

Symptoms may moderate over time, but the potential for an allergic reaction, once the right set of circumstances pops up, is always there. Once allergic, always allergic!

23.

Pitfalls to Avoid in Treatment

Ralph, eight, has the sort of moderate asthma that usually shows up with a respiratory infection. His condition seriously concerns his mother, who keeps going from one treatment approach to another in the hope of finding a "cure" for Ralph's wheezing. Over the past three years he has seen a chiropractor, an acupuncturist, and a psychic "healer" as well as the family doctor; he has taken a whole string of home remedies. One — consisting of a steaming hot mug of "natural" honey, lemon juice, and bourbon whiskey — made him very sleepy, impaired his breathing, and put him in the ER. He has swallowed massive doses of vitamins, minerals, and trace elements; he has briefly followed a succession of "free" diets; and he has eaten more "health" foods than one would believe possible. His symptoms remain unaffected.

Over the past 15 years a valuable series of studies has focused on the extent of and the reasons for nonadherence to treatment regimens for chronic conditions. These investigations have been extremely revealing. Even for moderate to severe chronic diseases (including allergic complaints), more than half of all patients fail to stick with the course of treatment prescribed by their physicians. Complete or partial nonadherence to what the doctor orders is the rule rather than the exception in patient behavior.

Why this massive failure to stick with medical recommendations? There are a number of factors involved, and they have to do with the complex interrelationships between physician, patient, the nature of the disease itself, and the treatment prescribed.

THE PHYSICIAN

The doctor is often at fault for a patient's failure to adhere to treatment. Some of the more common ways in which doctors promote nonadherence include failure to explain the nature of the disease or the treatment for it adequately; misdiagnosing the ailment; and prescribing inappropriate treatment. One shocking study revealed that, on the average, doctors spend less than 10 minutes treating patients with respiratory conditions. This is simply not enough time to do a competent and thorough examination and history, let alone make a sure diagnosis and explain what may be a complex, multifaceted treatment regimen.

Your responsibility as the parent of an allergic child is to insist, as is your right, that your physician take whatever time is necessary to assess your child's condition thoroughly. Be sure he or she explains the cause, nature, and course of the disease and its treatment in terms you fully understand. Your doctor should line out strategies for you to follow if treatment proves ineffectual ("If this doesn't clear up or gets worse in the next three or four days, call me") and recommend consultation if there are any problems or difficulties with either diagnosis or treatment.

THE PATIENT

Patients and care providers — parents — often have agendas that get in the way of effective treatment of allergic diseases in children. The ways that patients can fail to adhere to treatment are legion; the most prevalent ones include impatience with a slow rate of progress or improvement, over- or undermedicating, and "testing the limits."

Any chronic disease *taxes the patience* and good judgment of both the sick child and the parents. The disease wears on, the child improves slightly or not at all, tempers fray, and patience wears thin. Ultimately discouragement and frustration prompt parents to look to other sources of aid. And, with any chronic disease, allergies included, there is no shortage of alternative treatments — all of them certainly less effective than the up-to-date, advanced medical procedures we have described and many of them potentially hazardous for the patient.

These alternatives have one thing in common — they hold out hope; but it is a false hope, with disappointment and needless expense the payoff. While it is difficult to do, parents should reject the temptation to hop from one treatment to another. Chiropractors, herbalists, homeopaths, psychic "healers," and acupuncturists are not going to cure your child's allergies; mail order medications, home remedies, various kinds of exotic "tests" advertised in pulp magazines or junk mail flyers ("cytotoxic"; hair analysis) won't do it either. The pressure and the temptation to look to other such unorthodox forms of treatment is understandable. Resist it.

Over- or undermedicating are other forms of nonadherence to prescribed forms of treatment. In some allergic conditions — especially asthma — either one can be dangerous. *Undermedication* occurs in as many as 80% of the cases of children with moderate to severe asthma, usually when symptoms fade or go into remission. When the child appears to improve there is an understandable tendency to cut back, since administering medication can be time-consuming, messy, and emotionally taxing, as well as costly.

Overmedication when symptoms reappear or rebound stems from the popular fallacy that if a certain amount of medicine is good, more of it is better. Not only is this wrong, but, in the case of certain medicines used to treat respiratory allergies (Alupent or theophylline in particular), it can be hazardous or even lethal.

To avoid misuse of medication, parents should be absolutely clear on exactly how much medication their child should have and for how long a period. They need to be informed about negative side effects, know what to do should they occur, and know when to seek further advice if treatment fails or complications set in.

Related to the preceding points is the all-too-human tendency to *test the limits.* Once the allergic symptoms disappear or moderate, most people are tempted either to see if they can get along without the prescribed medication or to engage in forbidden activities. No one, children included, likes to be dependent on medication; most people do not relish having to think of themselves as limited in some way. They resent having to give up or forego a pleasurable activity that might provoke an allergic reaction.

"I wonder if I can get along without this darned Theo-dur?"

"Just a little helping of this shrimp dip shouldn't hurt me."

"The cat looks so lonely. Letting her in for just a short time shouldn't start me sneezing and wheezing."

Parents and children need to support one another and understand and accept the feelings of anger and frustration that accompany allergies and their treatment. Listening to one another, being aware of the likelihood of these feelings, and being honest in admitting to them lessens the temptation to pretend the condition no longer exists. Where anger, frustration, or denial persist, short-term counseling often proves to be a positive step. There are support groups designed to help individuals who have the condition or who are affected by those who have it.

MISUNDERSTANDING ALLERGIC DISEASE

Misunderstanding the nature of allergic disease causes problems, especially in cases of the chronic, more stubborn forms. In most instances the normal course of events is an allergy flares up, treatment is applied, and symptoms go away. We think the condition is gone for good because, ordinarily, there is no residual effect — the child appears completely normal, and there is usually no permanent damage. Gradually safeguards get suspended, and parents become less vigilant.

It is true that most (but not all) childhood allergic or hypersensitive reactions moderate with age (but not always). This leads parents to the belief that the child has "outgrown" the condition or is otherwise free of it. But for true allergies, the conditions that caused the original flare-up are always present; they are an ineradicable part of the genetic makeup of the child.

Remission of symptoms should not be taken as evidence of cure. At best, remission is a flight into health that, by assiduously avoiding triggers, one can prolong indefinitely. But the potential for another reaction, given the right set of circumstances, will accompany the allergic child always.

Another prominent and enormously damaging fable concerning allergic disease has to do with its cause. At one time it was thought that allergic disease was psychogenic, that is, psychologically rooted, with something in the individual's emotional life triggering the symptoms. This view prevailed in some scientific-medical circles for a period of about 20 years — until the mid 1960s when the role of IgE in allergy (especially the allergic triad of asthma, hay fever, and eczema) became absolutely clear and irrefutable. (Individual psychological factors can complicate allergies, as we discussed in Chapter 22, but they cannot *cause* them.) Still, belief in the unsubstantiated hypothesis that allergies grow out of psychological causes persists. Even some physicians (and many other uninformed or misinformed health care professionals including nurses, psychologists, and counselors) hold to it, and it is epidemic in the public at large.

In sum, *there is no persuasive evidence to support the contention that allergies are psychologically caused. Any treatment strategy founded on this belief will certainly turn out to be a costly failure.*

THE TREATMENT

The nature of the treatment itself is often enough to cause its own downfall. There are a number of ways this can happen.

1. *The treatment carries severe side effects.* For allergic diseases, these can range from drowsiness or torpor to severe respiratory or gastrointestinal complications. Physicians should but do not enumerate these, nor do they spell out what is to be done in the event of complications. Parents should demand this information; they can also inform themselves easily enough by consulting the *Physician's Desk Reference*, which is available in local libraries.

2. *The treatment is difficult or unpleasant.* Many of the medications, especially the ones for respiratory allergies, have an extremely unpleasant taste. Children will give Academy Award performances (including sobbing, retching, breath-holding, and other such displays) to avoid taking the drug. Most drugs do come in forms that can be ingested without the child having to taste it; ask the doctor for an alternative form if your child finds the medication difficult to get down.

Some treatments are abandoned because, in addition to being unpleasant, they are administered improperly and thus don't work. Inhalers are notoriously misused; some researchers have found that they are used ineffectively in three quarters of the cases. (See page 95 in Chapter 11 for the correct way to use an inhaler.)

Treatment may entail several medications' being taken according to a fixed time schedule and in a definite sequence. You, the parents, should be clear about the schedule and sequence, and see that it is carried out as ordered. If this is not done the whole process may be useless.

3. *The treatment is tedious and shows little or no apparent immediate gain.* This is true of some preventive measures like the breathing and diaphragm-strengthening exercises for asthma. Children (and adults, too) tire of such routine activities; they can be made more attractive, however, if you associate them with other pleasurable activities and make them as much like a game as possible.

4. *The treatment is essentially preventive in nature.* Medications like cromolyn (for asthma) or nasal steroids (for hay fever) have to be taken in the absence of symptoms or before symptoms are likely to occur. Children who feel well resist taking medication, partly because they see no valid reason for it. The connection needs to be explained to the child and the treatment, despite its apparent needlessness, enforced. Some parents find this authoritarian intervention difficult; if it is a problem for you, ask yourself whether you want a child who is resentful for a short period of time — or one who is sick and miserable.

5. *The treatment is expensive.* Some asthma and hay fever medications, especially, are quite expensive; often mere cost is enough to make parents cut back on or suspend dosage. Not only is this sort of economizing short lived, it can cause the child to develop a serious — and seriously expensive — condition.

24.

Vaccines and Immunization

Vaccines have virtually wiped out most common childhood diseases. They have done this by helping children (and adults, too) to develop an immunity that protects them from the disease-causing agent.

The general principle of immunization was hit upon by William Jenner, an English physician, almost 200 years ago. Jenner noticed that milkmaids, women who milked cows, were prone to develop cowpox, a mild skin infection, but almost never contracted smallpox, a deadly disease widely prevalent at that time. Jenner reasoned that cowpox (which the women contracted by coming in contact with the cows' udders) was a weak form of smallpox and that having it somehow made the milkmaids resistant to the killer disease. He then induced cowpox in well people by scratching their skin and introducing an extract from cows' udders into the wound. The result? The people treated in this way developed a mild case of cowpox but never got smallpox.

Smallpox, once one of the most dreaded of all diseases, was declared eradicated not too long ago; since Jenner's time vaccines have been developed to confer immunity to diphtheria, measles, mumps, pertussis (whooping cough), poliomyelitis, rubella (German measles), and tetanus. Other vaccines for special at-risk groups are available for tuberculosis, hepatitis, and pneumococcal pneumonia.

These vaccines have been marvelously effective. In this country, the combined number of reported cases of all these diseases has declined, in the past half-century, from over one million to fewer than 10,000 a year.

HOW IMMUNIZATION WORKS

Immunization is either *active* — stimulating the body to manufacture its own disease-fighting antibodies — or *passive* — administering preformed antibodies that confer temporary immunity. In the case of active immunization, either a vaccine or a toxoid is introduced. Vaccines contain killed or weakened disease organisms. Toxoids carry bacteria that have been made nontoxic; that is, they cannot trigger the disease but they can stimulate the body to produce its own antitoxins or antibodies. Preformed antibodies that confer passive immunity are usually derived from serum (blood), either human or animal.

In general, vaccines made from live, weakened microorganisms confer lifelong protection, and immunization needs only to be done once; in other forms of vaccines, booster shots may be required periodically.

IMMUNIZATION AND YOUR CHILD

Providing your child with a proper series of immunizations is a vital part of their health care; most states in the United States have laws that require schoolchildren to show evidence of vaccination before they are first enrolled. However, because *allergic* diseases either are linked to or are the outgrowth of immunological disorders, for allergic children, immunization presents special risks that need to be taken into account. You and your doctor should weigh the undoubted advantages of immunization procedures against the heightened risks they pose for some allergic children. The following sections summarize the vaccines employed for various diseases and their usual side effects and discuss any special problems or contraindications they represent for allergic youngsters. Information on vaccines can be obtained by calling your local Department of Public Health, or by writing or calling

Division of Immunization
Centers for Disease Control
1600 Clifton Road, N.E.
Atlanta, GA 30329
(404) 639-3311

Diphtheria, Tetanus, Pertussis (DTP)

WHEN AND FOR WHOM? The combined diphtheria, tetanus, pertussis vaccination is routinely recommended for all normal infants and children. It is usually given as a series of five injections according to the following schedule:

Age	*Immunization #*
2 months	1
4 months	2
6 months	3
18 months	4
4–6 years	5

Tetanus boosters alone are then recommended every 10 years or so; the first of these would be given at about age 14–16.

USUAL SIDE EFFECTS OF DTP. Each of the three components in the diphtheria, tetanus, pertussis vaccine has its own unique profile. The *diphtheria* vaccine is generally innocuous; few if any significant reactions to it have ever been reported. *Tetanus*, however, can cause significant local tenderness with muscle aches and pains around the site of the injection.

Of the three elements in DTP vaccine, the major offender is *pertussis*. Pertussis can produce swelling and pain at the injection site. Rarely, it can also lead to fever, convulsions, and even death. Pertussis vaccine has succeeded in virtually eliminating whooping cough in much of the world; it is an important and powerful public health tool. However, the pain and swelling is more than some parents want their children to endure. We suggest you discuss this with your physician. Generally, in normal children, we recommend routine use of pertussis vaccine, unless earlier reactions to the vaccines have been particularly troublesome.

DTP FOR ALLERGIC CHILDREN. Pertussis has a side effect that has been demonstrated experimentally; when animals are given the pertussis vaccine they often produce more of the IgE antibodies that generate allergies. Children who are atopic (see Chapter 1, pages 6 to 8) and already have a high incidence of allergies make far more IgE than they need. Thus, following administration of pertussis vaccine, their allergies may get significantly worse. For this reason we do not recommend pertussis vaccination in any child who has a history of moderate to severe hay fever, asthma, or eczema. (See Chapter 20, page 163 for more on the subject of whooping cough and vaccination against it.)

EFFECTIVENESS OF DTP. The DTP vaccine is remarkably effective. Diphtheria, tetanus, and pertussis have all but disappeared from our population; when outbreaks of them occur, they are almost always found only in children who have not been immunized.

Measles, Mumps, Rubella (MMR)

WHEN AND FOR WHOM? Containing live but weakened or attenuated viruses, MMR is administered as a combined vaccine. It is usually given at 15 months of age as a single, one-time immunization. The body makes an immune response to the weakened virus, which then protects against the real virus. The weakened virus is enough to induce an immune response, but it is not enough to cause significant disease. We recommend MMR for all normal children.

USUAL SIDE EFFECTS OF MMR. Live virus vaccines contain small numbers of the "bugs" that must divide and multiply in the body to induce the immune response. Therefore, reactions to all three of these live virus vaccines are not uncommon. *Measles* provides a good general example. In a significant number of children, mild fever and a slight rash *may* occur about 5–12 days following immunization.

MMR FOR ALLERGIC CHILDREN. MMR may be contraindicated if your child reacts to materials used in the laboratory to make the product. These materials may include egg proteins or antibiotics. For this reason, it is important that you let your doctor know if your child has any sensitivity to egg whites or antibiotics.

In addition, since a live virus is being administered, it is absolutely imperative that your child have normal immune function. Children whose immune systems are compromised — those born without a normal immune system, for example — may not be able to kill the attenuated viruses. This deficiency may even prove fatal. Most physicians are acutely aware of this possibility, and they treat such immune-compromised children so gingerly that virtually all of the parents know about the risk. However, they may *not* know that the live virus can spread from normal children to children with compromised immune systems.

Jeb has had reduced immune function all of his life from a rare disease known as DiGeorge syndrome. He was born without a completely normal thymus. He received a thymus transplant at birth and has done fairly well since, although he is still very susceptible to infections. When he was three years of age his sister Helen received her measles shot at 15 months as recommended. Helen did fine but about a week later Jeb began to show signs of severe, disseminated measles.

EFFECTIVENESS OF MMR. MMR has also been outstandingly effective. In the United States in 1949 there were over one million cases of measles, mumps, and rubella combined; in 1985 the total came to just over six thousand.

Poliomyelitis

WHEN AND FOR WHOM? Polio immunization is conferred through administration of an oral vaccine that contains weakened strains of polio virus types 1, 2, and 3. The viruses remain in the mouth, moving eventually to the gut and finally being excreted in the feces. The presence of the viruses in the gut is enough for the body to make a sufficient antibody response to safeguard the child.

The polio vaccine is administered according to the following schedule:

Age	*Immunization #*
2 months	1
4 months	2
18 months	3
4–6 years	4

We recommend completion of the polio vaccine series.

USUAL SIDE EFFECTS OF POLIO VACCINE. Polio vaccine almost never carries side effects; on extremely rare occasions the virus can mutate and become disease-causing again. This is an unlikely event, so rare it is best disregarded.

POLIO VACCINE FOR ALLERGIC CHILDREN. We urge polio vaccination for all except immunity-impaired children. Because live virus is carried in the stool, children with compromised immune function can receive the virus by coming in contact with the feces of other children or adults.

EFFECTIVENESS OF POLIO VACCINE. In 1952, the peak year for polio in the United States, 21,269 cases were reported; 1985 saw five cases.

Influenza

Influenza vaccines (flu shots) are relatively effective; however, since the form or type of the virus changes from year to year, the vaccines administered may not be specific to what's going round in any given year. The usual side effects are soreness and fever. Rarely, the vaccine may trigger Guillain-Barré syndrome, a progressive but reversible nerve paralysis that starts in the feet and ascends up the body.

There are no contraindications of flu shots for allergic children. Flu shots may not be effective for everyone; however, should influenza develop in an asthmatic child, the consequences could be quite serious, making the asthma much worse. On balance we advocate flu shots for asthmatic children; the potential benefits far outweigh the potential risks.

Pneumococcus

Pneumococcus vaccine protects against the bacteria that cause pneumonia. Most children have good immune systems and ward off this disease readily; even if it does develop, it responds quickly to antibiotics. Accordingly, the vaccine is not called for in most children, normal or allergic. However, children who have had their spleens removed or children with sickle cell anemia should receive this vaccine because their ability to combat pneumonia bacteria is impaired. (Sickle cell anemia is a blood disease found primarily in ethnic groups that have migrated to the U.S. from areas where malaria is endemic: Africa, the Mediterranean rim, and Central America.)

Hepatitis

There are two major types of hepatitis (liver) infections — A and B. *Hepatitis A*, the more common form, is generally spread by fecal contamination of foods. It is most often encountered in crowded, unsanitary living conditions, but it is relatively benign, of short duration, and has no significant side effects. Hepatitis A can be guarded against most effectively by observing good hygiene habits and avoiding foods susceptible to fecal contamination (seafoods, especially shellfish; certain other foods, depending on locale).

Gammaglobulin, an extract from the blood of healthy individuals who carry hepatitis A antibodies, also provides limited immunity. If you plan to travel to Central America, Asia, or Africa, gammaglobulin provides short-term (several months') protection against the hepatitis A virus and should be considered for all members of the family, allergic or not. (See also the section on gammaglobulin below.)

Hepatitis B, serum hepatitis, is a much more serious and stubborn disease. Sometimes fatal, it can cause extensive liver damage. It is most often spread through use or sharing of contaminated hypodermic needles or syringes or through blood transfusions; it is frequently encountered in intravenous drug users; it can also be transmitted sexually.

For ordinary individuals, the risk of contracting hepatitis B is slight, and vaccination for it is not routinely indicated. There is a hepatitis B vaccine available for use by individuals in high-risk groups — physicians and other health care providers who treat drug users or handle blood products.

Smallpox

Smallpox was declared eradicated a few years ago, and smallpox vaccinations are no longer routinely given to children. Even so, the disease still represents something of a danger. In order to guard our armed forces from the threat of biological warfare, all members of the military continue to receive smallpox vaccinations. As a result, every year a few newly vaccinated persons carry the weakened virus home, where children whose immune systems are in some way deficient come into contact with and contract the disease. Even more common is the spread of the virus to children with eczema. Skin with eczema is *very* susceptible to the virus in the vaccine; and *death* may even occur! So, ironically, the only real threat grows out of the vaccination procedures that did away with this once-virulent killer. The danger is, of course, minuscule, but if you are in the military and have a child with an impaired immune system or eczema, you should be aware of the remote possibility that the virus could be passed on. If your immunity-compromised child is in contact with military personnel or their children, check with your physician.

Other Vaccines

There are other vaccines not in widespread use and not ordinarily given to children: *plague, yellow fever, cholera, typhoid fever, tuberculosis, Rocky Mountain spotted fever, rabies*. For children, allergic or not, there are no special circumstances associated with these vaccines *except* that some of them are prepared or cultivated by using eggs. Here again, if your child is allergic to eggs, administration of one of the egg-grown vaccines could trigger a reaction. Alert your doctor to this possible complication as you work to achieve an optimal level of immunity in your children.

A NOTE ON GAMMAGLOBULIN

Gammaglobulin is the antibody-containing fraction of donor blood that is often useful in preventing infections. Children without the ability to make antibodies can be given shots once per month containing antibodies derived from healthy people. These shots are often enough to permit them to lead normal lives; without them they would die.

Doug is an 11-year-old with Bruton's syndrome. He was born without the ability to make antibodies. His younger brother Steve also had this disease. (It tends to run in males.) Before Doug was diagnosed as having Bruton's syndrome at age 18 months, he had recurrent bouts of pneumonia and ear infections. His doctor finally did a total serum antibody test and found that Doug had a major reduction in the normal antibody level. He has been receiving an injection of gammaglobulin every month since the discovery and has been virtually symptom-free.

Gammaglobulin has been used primarily in children like Doug who have congenital immune deficiency diseases. In fact, there has recently been a major improvement in the use of gammaglobulin — an intravenous preparation delivered directly into the blood of the recipient, rather than by intramuscular injection as was done formerly. The new preparation has fewer side effects and seems to work much better at preventing infections.

Gammaglobulin can also be used as a prophylactic in individuals who have been or are likely to be exposed to certain diseases — hepatitis A especially. If you or your children plan on traveling to a high-risk hepatitis area, it is often routinely recommended that you and they receive a hepatitis-preventive injection of gammaglobulin. The passive immunity that the injection confers by putting somebody else's antibodies to work will protect against hepatitis.

Ironically, the major side effect of gammaglobulin is an allergic reaction. Because you are receiving injections of protein from someone else you may make antibodies against it; this can result in swelling, fever, and enlargement of lymph nodes and spleen. It can even trigger an acute anaphylactic or shock reaction. If you have never experienced such a reaction before it is unlikely that it would occur, but the possibility does exist.

Gammaglobulin shots are extremely expensive so they are not likely to be given routinely. They are not usually recommended except under the special circumstances mentioned above.

A SPECIAL WORD FOR EXPECTANT MOTHERS

Live virus vaccinations are *never* recommended for women who are or who are trying to become pregnant; any vaccination at all during pregnancy should be discussed with your physician. The use of such vaccines, especially rubella (German measles), can significantly damage the fetus.

It is routinely recommended that all women of child-bearing age receive a blood test to see if they are immune to rubella. If they are not, then rubella vaccination should be administered at a time well in advance of any planned pregnancy. Being exposed to the attenuated rubella vaccine is just as injurious to the fetus as being nurtured by a mother with an actual case of German measles.

A NOTE ON THE NEEDLE

Vaccinations and other injections are immediately and sometimes sharply painful, and children quickly learn to associate this abrupt pain with visits to the doctor's office. When the child is told of an upcoming visit to the doctor, fear, dread, and even hysterical crying before and during the event can occur.

You can make things easier for both your child and the doctor by taking some simple precautionary steps.

1. Don't emphasize the fact that there may be a vaccination or injection.
2. NEVER use the threat of injection as a means of enforcing discipline at home. (It is surprising how many parents tell their children that if they don't behave they'll be taken to the doctor for a shot.)
3. If there is to be a shot, let the child know shortly in advance of the event that it will be given and why; whenever possible let the child make any of the decisions that don't need to be made by the doctor, for example, where the injection is to be made, and let the child share in the process to the fullest extent possible.
4. Treat injections as the ordinary, run-of-the-mill events they are. Avoid rebellious reactions or tantrums by reminding the child that the pain and discomfort are short-lived and by reinforcing cooperative and unafraid behavior.
5. If your child reacts strongly to injections, let the doctor know in advance so that he or she can be prepared. Advise the doctor concerning any strategies you know of that keep your child relatively calm or quiescent.

Getting children to the point where they accept injections (and blood drawing) as routine aspects of medical care carries a number of important advantages for parents, physician, and child.

For some allergic children, asthmatics and those with eczema in particular, the intense emotional reaction to the needle can provoke or intensify symptoms. In other children who have serious conditioned fear reactions, the actual injection or the mere sight of the needle can bring about a vascular collapse, with dizziness, fainting, or even more severe consequences.

ALLERGY SHOTS

A special type of vaccine, commonly known as allergy shots or immunotherapy, is the injection of extracts prepared from allergens. The only people who should receive allergy shots are those who clearly have IgE-mediated disease, as revealed by skin tests and a clear history. In most instances, a physician can predict by the patient's history whether the symptoms justify the allergy shots or not. Just because someone has positive skin tests does not mean that he or she would be helped by shots.

Allergy shots are made up of a dilute mixture of the allergens the patient is allergic to. Thereafter, once or twice a week, the patient receives an injection in the arm. With each visit, and assuming there is no bad reaction, the dose of the shot is increased. Following each injection, the patient must stay in the doctor's office for at least 30 minutes in case he or she shows signs of a local or a systemic reaction. A local reaction can be as mild as some warmth at the injection site or as severe as very bad swelling and pain. A systemic reaction can include shortness of breath, wheezing, hives, and even shock. It is for these reasons that your doctor will observe your child for 30 minutes. If a mild reaction develops, the doctor is likely to decrease the dose of shots before proceeding to higher strengths.

The major reason for shots are allergies to common environmental agents such as house dust and pollens. Sometimes injections of molds are given, but the data on this procedure are poor, and they are not recommended until further research is done. Allergy shots to counteract sensitivity to pets are only recommended when an individual, such as a veterinarian, must be exposed to animals. Families who insist on allergy injections in preference to giving up their pets are sometimes accommodated, but the injections are risky, expensive, prolonged, and frequently ineffectual.

Chapters 11 to 15 discuss the role of allergy shots in specific problems with children. In general, the major indications are for allergic asthma that is not entirely controlled by pharmacotherapy and for airborne allergies that mediate hay fever and allergic conjunctivitis. As noted above, we never recommend allergy shots for patients with eczema, and it is very rare to manage hives with shots. In contrast, patients who have life-threatening allergies to insect stings are often very well controlled by injection of insect venom. Finally, we do not recommend the use of allergy shots for food allergy.

25.

The Long Haul: What Happens to Children with Allergies?

Thirty years ago, if a child had an allergy, he or she was pretty much stuck with it. Hay fever sufferers could sometimes be desensitized by going through a course of shots of dubious efficacy; persons having severe breathing problems brought on by an acute asthma attack could be helped temporarily by being injected with epinephrine. Then, in all likelihood, they would be referred to a psychiatrist. Effective medications to prevent or control the outbreak of allergic symptoms were all but unknown.

Since that time immense strides have been made in understanding the mechanisms of allergic disease, and, as a corollary to that understanding, various kinds of medications have appeared. We now have an impressive and effective array of allergy drugs — antihistamines, steroids, inhalants, and medications — that combat or forestall symptoms.

Even so, the underlying mechanisms of allergic or hypersensitive reactions are still not well or completely understood. As the biophysiology and biochemistry of allergic reactions come to be more fully known, as they certainly shall, and distinctions between the various forms of allergic disease become more clear-cut, even greater progress will be made in developing strategies and remedies that will allow easy management of these diseases.

Along with the improved medical management of symptoms, substantial progress has been made in the ability to avoid or control allergy-causing substances. Labeling requirements oblige manufacturers to tell us what their processed foods contain, thus permitting allergy-prone individuals to avoid some possible sources of trouble. There are still wide areas that need attention, of course; "fresh" foods, fruits and vegetables, are, in many instances, not required to carry labels naming the preservatives, insecticides, herbicides, or fungicides they have been treated with and are often contaminated by. (For instance, sulfites as preservatives on fresh fruits and vegetables were outlawed in January, 1987; however, the ban does not extend to potatoes or seafood, and the Environmental Protection Agency allows sulfites on fresh grapes provided 40% of the bunches carry warning labels. Users naturally assume that the unlabeled bunches are sulfite-free.) Nor do meats, poultry, fish, and shellfish packages have to list the preservatives, dyes, or antibiotics that may have invaded them.

As knowledge and concern over the extent to which chemicals have invaded our lives mounts, the supply of goods that have been produced with the intent of avoiding chemical contamination also grows. The chemical threat to health and well-being is being countered to a modest extent by the increased availability of contaminant-free products.

Along with the more precise information about what causes allergies and the development of effective medications to treat them has been an impressive improvement in the efficacy of devices to control the environment. The ability to control air temperature and purity efficiently has been a boon to many allergy sufferers.

There has also been a surge in self-management of symptoms. This move in the direction of self-care has heightened awareness of allergic symptoms and their triggers, and promises to make their management more judicious and effective.

These developments all argue the fact that, while allergies will continue to appear in a significant proportion of all children, their symptoms are likely to be less severe and persistent in years to come. There will be just as many allergic children in coming generations, but with the growth in knowledge about the nature of allergic diseases and the radically improved means of treating them, the symptoms will not be as debilitating and costly as they are today.

That is the long haul. What is the outlook for children who have allergic diseases right now? First, even under today's conditions, the long-term outlook for most children with allergic diseases is quite favorable. What happens during the process of maturation has a great deal to do with that bright prospect. Asthma and eczema usually moderate as the child grows older; only in a small minority of cases do they continue to be a problem into adulthood. Gastrointestinal difficulties also mostly disappear as the digestive apparatus matures. Hives are inclined to be much more prevalent in youngsters, although the reason for this is not clearly understood.

Hay fever and allergic contact dermatitis (ACD) are exceptions to the general rule that allergies ease off with age. Both hay fever and ACD require a period of sensitization before they show. Once the child is sensitized the symptoms are likely to persist and to become worse over time, but the good news here is that there are extremely effective preventive medications to combat hay fever, and ACD can be readily controlled by keeping away from whatever it is that triggers the rash.

Not only does growing up help to lighten allergic symptoms; it also eases some of the nonallergic difficulties brought on by allergies. Chronic earache or eye problems usually abate by the time the child reaches six years of age.

Not only do symptoms usually fade away gradually; when they vanish they carry their signs with them. Asthmatics will not suffer permanent lung damage. The skin recovers, unblemished, from eczema, hives, or contact dermatitis. Most children are likely to escape completely physically unscathed from their allergic experiences.

This should not encourage you to believe that childhood allergies are nothing more than a passing nuisance. For many — perhaps most — they are, but for some kids they amount to considerably more than that. In a small percentage of instances the condition can be life-threatening, especially in the case of asthma or acute sensitivity reactions to things like food and food additives, antibiotics, and insect stings and bites. And the incidence of asthma-related deaths in children seems to be on the rise. Although, as studies indicate, the reasons for the increase are complex and many-faceted, simple disregard of symptoms, under-medication, and psychological depression are prominent among them. Significantly, all of these factors are more closely tied to the home than to hospital or clinic.

Some children do carry their allergies into adult life. Hay fever and allergic contact dermatitis, as noted, are likely to have lifelong runs; asthma, eczema, and hives can also persist for a lifetime. Even so, when they do tag along into adulthood, the symptoms can usually be managed by observing a few precautions and by sticking with prescribed medication. Most allergic adults are able to get along with reasonable comfort and with no awkward limits placed on the range or level of their activities.

Among the potentially most damaging consequences of allergic disease is its psychological impact on affected children. Throughout the book we have emphasized the importance of having the allergic child lead a life as close as possible to normal, and we have suggested how he or she can be helped to do this. We have seen how often allergies lead parents to shield the child not only from the consequences of allergy, but from many of the good, enjoyable, fun parts of growing up. Such overprotection can have substantial and long-lasting effects on the child's personality and attitudes, undermining independence and self-reliance and creating dependency and a negative self-image. While it is true that there may be risks involved in having some allergic children participate in some aspects of the usual run of childhood activities, parents all too often lose sight of the fact that denying the child those experiences carries its own set of potential problems.

In summary, then, the long-range prognosis for your allergic child is upbeat. The chances are good that he or she will outgrow the symptoms or, if they do persist, the symptoms will probably be avoidable or manageable, even under today's conditions. They will certainly be more so as the nature of allergic disease and hyperreactivity comes to be more fully revealed in the next few years.

As parent you can best help in the development of your allergic child by trying to see to it that the youngster

- has knowledgeable, competent, and understanding care;
- participates fully and freely in as many of the ordinary aspects of growing up as can be managed; and
- is treated matter-of-factly, so that the disease does not become an excuse or an occasion for stunting his or her physical, psychological, or social development.

APPENDIX A

An Elimination Diet

Eat and drink only the foods listed below. All fruits and vegetables, except lettuce, must be cooked, or canned

Grains and Cereals

Rice
Rice wafers
Puffed rice, Rice flakes, Rice Krispies

Fruits

Apricots
Cranberries
Peaches
Pears

Meat

Lamb

Beverage

Water

Vegetables

Beets
Carrots
Chard
Lettuce
Oyster plant
Sweet potato

Oils and Seasoning

Olive oil, Crisco, Spry
Any vegetable oil (except oleomargarine)
Acetic acid vinegar (white)
Salt
Sugar (cane and beet)
Vanilla extract (synthetic)

Dessert

Tapioca

Suggested Menu:

Breakfast	*Lunch*	*Dinner*
Rice Krispies	Lamb chop	Lamb patty
Rice wafers	Sweet potato	Boiled rice
Peaches	Beets	Carrots
Apricot juice	Rice wafers	Lettuce with white vinegar
Peach jam	Cranberry juice	Peaches
Water	Pears	Apricot juice

AVOID: Coffee, tea, Coca Cola and other soft drinks, chewing gum, all medications except those ordered by a doctor.

INSTRUCTIONS: Stay on the basic diet for l4 days. If there are no changes in symptoms, stop the diet. But if the diet seems to be working,

- on day 15 add yellow vegetables all by themselves.
- on day 22 add green vegetables all by themselves.
- on day 31 add chicken all by itself.

Continue adding food groups one at a time at seven-day intervals. Keep a written record of what foods are added, when they are added, and the reaction, if any, to them. Add foods in large amounts, and eat them several times a day during addition period. If a reaction does occur, drop the newly added food or food group, return to the preceding week's diet, stay with it for a seven-day period, then reintroduce the food or food group associated with the reaction. If the reaction reappears, you have identified one cause or agent. Eliminate that food from the diet and continue adding foods as before until the process is completed.

APPENDIX B

Food Groupings

1. Apple — apple, pear, quince
2. Aster — lettuce, chicory, endive, escarole, artichoke, dandelion, sunflower seeds
3. Beet — beet, spinach, chard
4. Blueberry — blueberry, huckleberry, cranberry
5. Buckwheat — buckwheat, rhubarb, garden sorrel
6. Cashew — cashew, pistachio, mango
7. Chocolate — chocolate (cocoa), cola
8. Citrus — orange, lemon, grapefruit, lime, tangerine, kumquat, citron
9. Fungus — mushroom, yeast
10. Ginger — ginger, cardamom, turmeric
11. Gooseberry — gooseberry, currant
12. Grain (cereal or grass) — wheat, corn, rice, oats, barley, rye. Also wild rice, cane, millet, sorghum, bamboo shoots.
13. Laurel — avocado, cinnamon, bay leaves, sassafras
14. Mallow — cottonseed, okra
15. Melon (gourd) — watermelon, cucumber, cantaloupe, pumpkin, squash, other melons.
16. Mint — mint, peppermint, spearmint, thyme, sage, basil, savory, rosemary, catnip
17. Mustard — mustard, turnip, radish, horseradish, watercress, cabbage, sauerkraut, Chinese cabbage, broccoli, cauliflower, brussels sprouts, collards, kale, kohlrabi, rutabaga
18. Myrtle — allspice, guava, clove pimento (not pimento)

19. Onion — onion, garlic, asparagus, chives, leeks, sarsaparilla
20. Palm — coconut, date
21. Parsley — parsley, carrot, parsnip, celery, celeriac, anise, dill, fennel, angelica, celery seed, cumin, coriander, caraway
22. Pea (legume or clover) — peas (green, field, black-eyed), peanuts, beans (navy, lima, pinto, string, soy, etc.), licorice, acacia, tragacanth
23. Plum — plum, cherry, peach, apricot, nectarine, almond
24. Potato — potato, tomato, eggplant, green pepper, red pepper, chili pepper, paprika, cayenne
25. Rose — strawberry, raspberry, blackberry, dewberry, loganberry, youngberry, boysenberry
26. Walnut — English walnut, black walnut, pecan, hickory nut, butternut

APPENDIX C-1

Milk-Free Diet

Eliminate

Milk, including low-fat, skim, and buttermilk
Dairy products, including
- butter
- ice cream and sherbet
- all cheeses
- yogurt
- cottage cheese
- sour cream

Common foods that contain dairy products, such as
- puddings
- custards
- cream soups
- breads
- pastry
- spaghetti

All foods that contain (read labels)
- non-fat dry milk solids
- sodium (Na) caseinate
- whey

Chocolate, cocoa

APPENDIX C-2

Cereal-Free Diet

Foods Allowed

Starches
Tapioca
White potato
Sweet potato or yam
Soybean potato bread
Lima bean potato bread
Soybean milk

Meats
Lamb
Beef
Chicken, fryers, roasters
Capon (no hens)
Bacon
Liver (lamb)

Vegetables and Fruit
Artichoke
Asparagus
Beets
Carrots
Chard
Lettuce
Lima beans
Peas
Spinach
Squash
String beans
Tomato
Apricots
Grapefruit*
Lemon
Peaches
Pineapple
Prunes
Pears

Preservatives, etc.
Sugar, cane or beet
Salt
Sesame oil
Soybean oil
Willow Run oleomargarine
Gelatin (Knox's), flavored with allowed fruits and juices
Maple syrup or syrup made with cane sugar flavored with maple
White vinegar
Vanilla extract
Lemon extract
Corn-free baking powder
Baking soda
Cream of tartar

---

*The canned fruits should be preserved with cane sugar, not corn sugar. Water-packed fruits may be used and sweetened with cane sugar syrup.

APPENDIX D-I

Tyramine-Free Diet

Eliminate

Chocolate, cocoa, fava beans
All ripened cheeses
Avocados
Bananas
Canned figs
Fermented sausage (e.g., bologna, salami, pepperoni, aged beef, hot dogs)
Red wine, sherry
Beer
Chicken livers
Pickled herring
Anchovies
Dried fish
Yeast extracts

APPENDIX D-2

Salicylate-Free Diet

Eliminate

1. Foods

Almonds
Apples
Apricots
Blackberries
Cherries
Cucumbers and pickles
Currants
Gooseberries
Grapes and raisins
Nectarines
Oranges
Peaches
Plums and prunes
Raspberries
Strawberries
Tomatoes

2. Flavorings (artificially flavored and colored foods and drinks)

Breakfast cereals with artificial coloring and flavoring
Ice cream
Oleomargarine
Cake mixes
Bakery goods (except plain bread)
Jello (gelatin)
Licorice
Mint flavors
Oil of wintergreen
Jams and jellies
Lunch meats (salami, bologna, etc.)
Hot dogs

3. Beverages

Cider and cider vinegars
Wine and wine vinegars
Gin and all distilled drinks (except vodka)

Kool-Aid and similar beverages
Soda pop (all soft drinks)
Diet drinks and supplements
All tea
Beer

4. Drugs and miscellaneous

All medicines containing aspirin, such as Bufferin, Anacin, Excedrin, Alka-Seltzer, Empirin, Darvon compounds, etc.
Perfumes
Lozenges
Mouthwash
Toothpaste and toothpowder (baking soda can be used as a substitute)

Note: Check all labels of prepared foods and drugs for artificial flavorings or coloring.

Foods Allowed

1. All meats (except those that are artificially flavored, such as hot dogs, bologna, etc.)
2. All fish (except fish sticks)
3. Eggs
4. Milk and milk products
5. Butter or Willow Run margarine (purchase at health food stores)
6. All vegetables (except cucumbers and tomatoes)
7. All starches — plain bread, rice, potato, pancake mixes without coloring
8. Fruit — grapefruit, lemons, pears, bananas, dates, limes, figs
9. Beverages — coffee and Seven-Up
10. Others — pure maple syrup, all vegetable oils, distilled white vinegar, salt and pepper

Note: Tylenol may be used for fever or pain (purchase at a pharmacy).

APPENDIX D-3

Mold-Free Diet

Eliminate

All cheeses, including cottage cheese, sour cream, sour milk, buttermilk
Beer and wine
Cider and homemade root beer
Mushrooms
Soy sauce
Canned tomatoes, unless homemade
Pickled and smoked fish and meats, including sausages, hot dogs, corned beef, pastrami, pickled tongue
Vinegar and vinegar-containing foods, such as mayonnaise, pickles, pickled vegetables, green olives, sauerkraut
Soured breads (e.g., pumpernickel), fresh rolls, coffee cakes, other foods made with large amounts of yeast
All dried and candied fruits including raisins, apricots, dates, prunes, figs
Melons, especially cantaloupe

APPENDIX D-4

Foods and Other Materials Containing Tartrazine

Tartrazine is a dye (FD&C yellow #5) added to foods to "improve" their appearance. The list below is only suggestive of the literally thousands of places it may turn up. Read labels carefully. A typical label may read as follows:

"INGREDIENTS: Enriched wheat flour . . . whole wheat flour . . . oil shortening . . . sugar, corn syrup, salt, malted barley flour, lecithin, *FD&C yellow #5*, and artificial color."

Baked goods, bread with food dyes added, sweet breads, whole wheat
Butter
Candies
Cereals, colored
Cheeses
Chips (potato, corn, taco)
Fish, frozen (some; check label)
Fruits, canned (some; check label)
Ice creams
Jello (gelatin)
Lozenges
Margarine
Meats, prepared
Mouthwash
Mustard
Pudding
Sauces and gravies, prepared
Toothpaste
Yogurt

APPENDIX D-5

Foods and Other Materials Containing Sulfiting Agents

Metabisulfite (sodium bisulfite) is a food preservative and freshener. It is commonly used to keep prepared potatoes white (beware of fast-food french fries) and, until recently, was sprinkled on trays of ingredients at salad bars to maintain their appearance of freshness. It also turns up in many processed foods and beverages, including beer and wine. Here is a typical label for a product containing metabisulfite.

"INGREDIENTS: Cauliflower, vinegar, salt, dill, alum, and *sodium bisulfite*."

Beer
Cheeses
Cider
Cordials
Fruit juices
Glucose (syrup and solid)
Jello (gelatin)
Pickles
Potatoes, whole, peeled, or sliced (raw)
Sausages and sausage meat
Vegetables, dehydrated (especially peas)
Vinegar
Wines (red, white, or rosé)

APPENDIX E

Pollen Map and Guide for the United States*

Map Area	*Trees*[1]	*Grasses*[2]	*Weeds*[3]
I CT, ME, MA, NH, NJ, NY, PA, RI, VT	Maple/Box Elder Oak Birch	Timothy Orchard Fescue Redtop	Lamb's-quarter Ragweed, giant & short Cocklebur
II DE, DC, MD, NC, VA	Maple/Box Elder Birch Juniper/Cedar	Redtop Vernal grass Bermuda grass Orchard grass Timothy	Pigweed Lamb's-quarter Ragweed, giant & short Mexican fire bush
III FL (North), GA, SC	Maple/Box Elder Birch Juniper/Cedar	Redtop Vernal grass Bermuda grass Orchard grass Rye grass	Lamb's-quarter Ragweed, giant & short Sagebrush English plantain
IV FL (South)	Box Elder Oak Juniper/Cedar	Redtop Bermuda grass Salt grass Bahia grass	Pigweed Lamb's-quarter Ragweed, giant & short Sagebrush
V IN, KY, OH, TN, WV	Maple/Box Elder Birch Oak Hickory	Redtop Bermuda grass Orchard grass Fescue Rye grass	Waterhemp Pigweed Lamb's-quarter Ragweed, giant & short

[1]Pollenating season ordinarily late winter through spring.
[2]Pollenating season ordinarily spring through early summer.
[3]Pollenating season ordinarily summer through early fall.
*Only the more common and widespread pollens for each area are listed.

Map Area	*Trees*	*Grasses*	*Weeds*
VI AL, AR, LA, MI	Maple/Box Elder Juniper/Cedar Oak	Redtop Bermuda grass Orchard grass Rye grass Timothy	Carelessweed/Pigweed Lamb's-quarter Ragweed, giant & short
VII MI, MN, WI	Maple/Box Elder Alder Birch Oak	Redtop Brome Orchard grass Fescue Rye grass	Waterhemp Lamb's-quarter Russian thistle Ragweed, giant & short
VIII IL, IA, MO	Maple/Box Elder Birch Oak Hickory	Redtop Bermuda grass Orchard grass Rye grass Timothy	Pigweed Lamb's-quarter Mexican fire bush Russian thistle Ragweed, giant, & short
IX KA,NB,ND,SD	Maple/Box Elder Alder Birch Hazelnut Oak	Quack grass/Wheat grass Redtop Brome Orchard grass Rye grass	Waterhemp Pigweed Lamb's-quarter Mexican fire bush Russian thistle Ragweed, false, giant, short & western
X OK, TX	Box Elder Juniper/Cedar Oak Mesquite	Quack grass/Wheat grass Redtop Bermuda grass Orchard grass	Waterhemp Carelessweed/Pigweed Saltbush/Scale Lamb's-quarter
XI AZ, CO, ID, MT, NM, UT, WY	Box Elder Alder Birch Juniper/Cedar Oak	Quack grass/Wheat grass Redtop Brome Bermuda grass Orchard grass	Waterhemp Pigweed Saltbush/Scale Sugarbeet Lamb's-quarter Mexican fire bush
XII AZ (Desert), CA (Southeastern Desert)	Cypress Juniper/Cedar Mesquite Ash Olive	Brome Bermuda grass Salt grass Rye grass Canary grass June grass	Carelessweed Iodine bush Saltbush/Scale Lamb's-quarter Russian thistle Ragweed, false, slender, & western

Map Area	*Trees*	*Grasses*	*Weeds*
XIII CA (Southern coastal)	Box Elder Cypress Oak Walnut Acacia	Oats Brome Bermuda grass Orchard grass Salt grass	Carelessweed/Pigweed Saltbush/Scale Lamb's-quarter Russian thistle Ragweed, false, slender, & western
XIV CA (Central valley)	Box Elder Alder Birch Cypress Oak Pecan	Redtop Oats Brome Bermuda grass Rye grass Orchard grass	Pigweed Saltbush/Scale Sugarbeet Lamb's-quarter Russian thistle Ragweed, false, slender, & western
XV ID (southern), NE	Box Elder Alder Birch Juniper/Cedar Ash	Quack grass/Wheat grass Redtop Brome Bermuda grass Orchard grass	Pigweed Iodine bush Saltbush/Scale Lamb's-quarter Mexican fire bush Russian thistle
XVI OR Central & Eastern), WA (Central & Eastern)	Box Elder Alder Birch Oak Walnut Pine	Quack grass/Wheat grass Redtop Vernal grass Brome Orchard grass	Pigweed Saltbush/Scale Lamb's-quarter Mexican fire bush Russian thistle Ragweed, false, giant, short, & western
XVII CA (Northwestern), WA (Western), OR (Western)	Box Elder Alder Birch Hazelnut Oak Walnut Ash	Bent grass Vernal grass Oats Brome Bermuda grass Orchard grass Salt grass	Pigweed Saltbush/Scale Lamb's-quarter Russian thistle Ragweed, false, giant, short, & western
ALASKA	Alder Aspen Birch Cedar Hemlock	Blue grass/June grass Brome Canary grass Fescue	Bullrush Dock/Sorrel Lamb's-quarter Nettle Plantain
HAWAII	Acacia Beefwood Juniper/Cedar Cypress	Bermuda grass Corn Finger grass Johnson grass Love grass	Cocklebur Plantain Kochia Pigweed Ragweed, slender

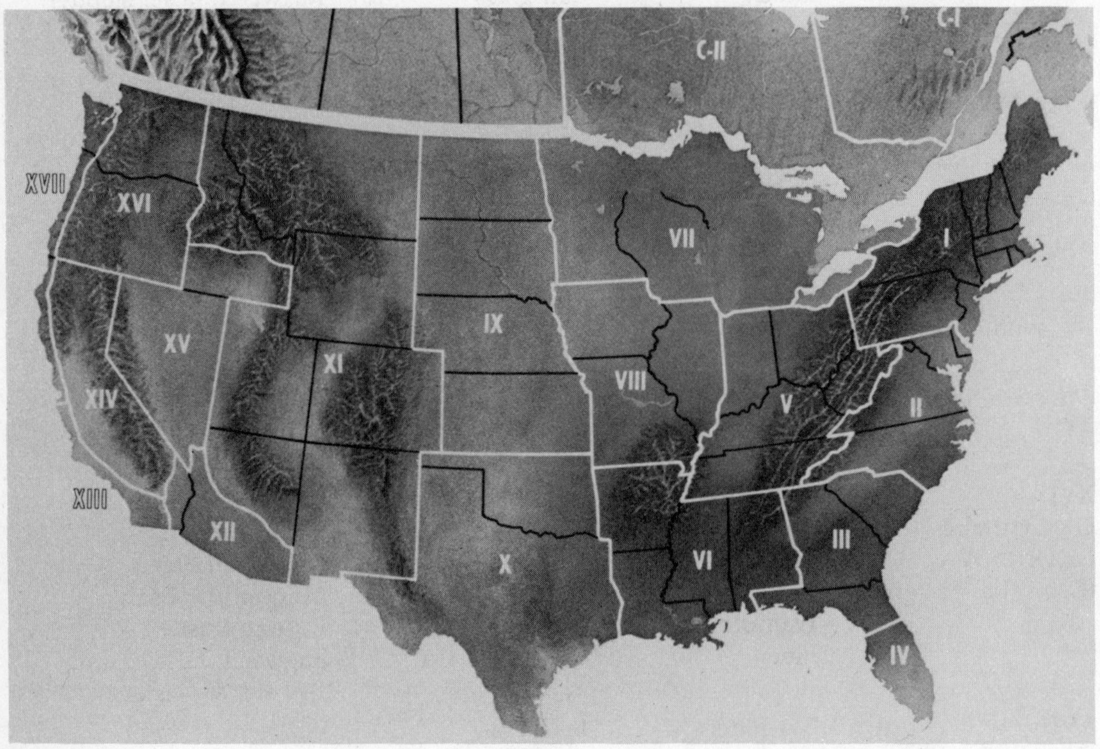

This botanical region map of the United States is reproduced with permission of Miles Pharmaceutical Division, West Haven, CT. It is reproduced from *Botanical Regions of the United States and Canada*, 1975.

APPENDIX F

Air Filtration Devices

Suppliers of air filtration devices are listed under "Air Cleaning and Purifying Equipment" in the classified section of the telephone directory.

There are three main kinds of filtration equipment, and they are classified according to the type of filter. Some use electrostatic or electronic filters; others have fine screens that trap dust or pollen; still others ionize particles, giving them a negative electrical charge that causes them to attach to positively charged surfaces.

Each type of device has a large number of manufacturers, and their products vary greatly in size, price, quality, and efficacy. If you decide to get air filtration equipment, keep the following points in mind.

1. Medical supply firms (also listed in the Yellow Pages) stock an inventory of these devices. Some allow customers to try out units prior to rental or purchase. Ask if this is possible. If not, rent for a trial period. *Try before buying!*
2. To be effective, a room-sized purifier should recirculate the air at least four times per hour. Thus, a unit to be placed in a 12 × 15 foot room (with the conventional 8-foot ceiling) would have to have a rated capacity of not less than 100 cubic feet per minute (c.f.m.). To calculate the size of unit needed, multiply the volume of the room in cubic feet (length × width × height) by 4 and then divide that result by 60.
3. Tightly fitting window filters that act to screen out larger airborne particles are a useful adjunct to purifiers.

4. Pay close attention to the specifications of the equipment you rent or purchase, and monitor your child's symptoms before and after the unit is put in service. There are a large number of units that do little or nothing to improve air quality, and some of them that produce a large amount of ozone actually degrade it.
5. Tabled below are typical rental and purchase costs, maintenance features, and general comments about each of these types of air purifiers.

Filter Type	*Purchase Price*	*Monthly Rental*	*Filter Costs*	*Maintenance*	*Comment*
Electronic or electrostatic	$300 and up	$40 and up	N/A	Wash filter regularly	Some noise; some brands produce unacceptably high levels of ozone, an irritant
HEPA (High Efficiency Particulate Arresting)	$400 and up	$50 and up	$40–$80	Replace filter screen every 18 months	Some noise; over a 5-year period cost an estimated 50% more than comparably priced electrostatic unit
Fiber	$100 and up	$15 and up	$5–$20	Replace filter screen monthly	Some noise; nat as efficient as HEPA; some models ineffective
Ionizing	Up to $100	Up to $15	N/A	Clean surfaces attracting negatively charged particles	Quiet; units small, more than one needed for large space; some models ineffective

Note: Some units may incorporate a variety of filters or traps; others employ activated charcoal pads which remove tobacco smoke.

For a central unit we recommend the Newtron. Newtron Products, 3874 Virginia Avenue, P.O. Box 27175, Cincinnati, OH 45227 (800-543-9149).

The Association of Home Appliance Manufacturers, 20 North Wacker Drive, Chicago, IL 60606, has a list of certified room air cleaners. Write them for their up-to-date recommendations and the specifications of the units they certify.

APPENDIX G

Summer Camps for Allergic (Asthmatic) Children

Camps for allergic and asthmatic children come and go, dependent as they are on community interest and support. Listed below, alphabetically by state, are localities that have regularly offered such camps and the organizations or agencies sponsoring them.

To learn about such camps in your area, call your local chapter of the American Lung Association (ALA). It will be listed in the white pages of the telephone directory.

Communities Offering Camps for Asthmatic Children, by Sponsoring Organization and State

Arizona

Arizona Asthma Foundation
Glendale, Arizona
(602) 938-1383

Arkansas

American Lung Association
Little Rock, Arkansas
(501) 374-3726

California

American Lung Association
Fresno, California
(800) 367-5864

American Lung Association
Los Angeles, California
(213) 935-5864

American Lung Association
Contra Costa/Solano Counties
(415) 935-0472

American Lung Association
Santa Ana, California
(714) 835-5864

American Lung Association
San Diego, California
(619) 297-3901

American Lung Association
San Francisco, California
(415) 543-4410

American Lung Association
San Mateo, California
(415) 349-1111

American Lung Association
Oakland, California
(415) 893-5474

Asthma and Allergy Foundation of America
Los Angeles, California
(213) 937-7859

Colorado

American Lung Association
Pueblo, Colorado
(303) 543-5864

Colorado Allergy Society
Englewood, Colorado
(303) 232-1428

Florida

American Lung Association
Fort Lauderdale, Florida
(305) 524-4657

American Lung Association
Jacksonville, Florida
(904) 743-2933

Georgia

American Lung Association
Atlanta, Georgia
(404) 872-9653

Illinois

Asthma and Allergy Foundation of America
Chicago, Illinois
(312) 346-0745

Indiana

American Lung Association
Indianapolis, Indiana
(317) 872-9685

Iowa

American Lung Association
Des Moines, Iowa
(515) 243-1225

Kansas

American Lung Association
Overland Park, Kansas
(913) 648-0688

Maine

American Lung Association
Augusta, Maine
(207) 622-6394

Massachusetts

American Lung Association
Topsfield, Massachusetts
(617) 887-6055

Michigan

American Lung Association
Lansing, Michigan
(517) 484-4541

American Lung Association
Southfield, Michigan
(313) 559-5100

Minnesota

American Lung Association
Minneapolis, Minnesota
(612) 871-7332

Montana

American Lung Association
Helena, Montana
(406) 442-6556

Nebraska

American Lung Association
Omaha, Nebraska
(402) 393-2222

New Hampshire

American Lung Association
Manchester, New Hampshire
(603) 669-2411

New Mexico

American Lung Association
Alberquerque, New Mexico
(505) 265-0732

New York

American Lung Association
Utica, New York
(315) 735-9225

American Lung Association
New York City, New York
(212) 889-3370

North Dakota

American Lung Association
Bismarck, North Dakota
(701) 223-5613

Ohio

American Lung Association
Cincinnati, Ohio
(513) 751-3650

Oklahoma

American Lung Association
Tulsa, Oklahoma
(918) 747-3441

Oregon

American Lung Association
Portland, Oregon
(503) 224-5145

Virginia

Camp Holiday Trails (Private)
Charlottesville, Virginia
(804) 977-3781

Washington

American Lung Association
Seattle, Washington
(206) 441-5100

Children's Orthopedic Hospital
Seattle, Washington
(206) 526-2000

APPENDIX H

Organizations Concerned with Allergy Information or Treatment Programs

American Academy of Allergy and Immunology
611 East Wells Street
Milwaukee, WI 53202

American Allergy Association
P.O. Box 7273
Menlo Park, CA 94026

American Lung Association
1740 Broadway
New York, NY 10036

Asthma and Allergy Foundation of America
1302 18th Street, N.W., Suite 30
Washington, DC 20036

Asthma Project,
National Heart, Lung, and Blood Institute
Building 31, Room 4A-21
Bethesda, MD 20205

National Foundation for Asthma
P.O. Box 50304
Tucson, AZ 85703

National Institute of Allergy and Infectious Diseases
National Institutes of Health
Bethesda, MD 20205

APPENDIX I

Allergy Centers and Clinics

Listed below, alphabetically by state and city, are many of the major allergy centers and clinics at hospitals throughout the country. These clinics offer advanced outpatient care for allergy sufferers. Other allergy clinics may be located through your Health Maintenance Organization, allergist, the allergy department of a nearby teaching hospital or university medical school, or your local American Lung Association chapter.

Arkansas

University of Arkansas Medical Center
4301 W. Markham Street
Little Rock, AR 72201
(501) 661-5000

California

Scripps Clinic and Research Foundation
476 Prospect Street
La Jolla, CA 92037
(714) 455-9100

Los Angeles–USC Medical Center
1200 N. State Street
Los Angeles, CA 90033
(213) 226-6503

UCLA Hospital
10833 Le Conte Avenue
Los Angeles, CA 90024
(213) 825-6481

University of California, Irvine, Medical Center
101 City Drive South
Orange, CA 92668
(714) 634-6011

Children's Hospital at Stanford
520 Willow Road
Palo Alto, CA 94304
(415) 327-4800

University of California Medical Center
2315 Stockton Blvd.
Sacramento, CA 95817
(916) 453-3737

University Hospital
University of California Medical Center
225 W. Dickinson Street
San Diego, CA 92103
(714) 294-6222

Kaiser Foundation Hospital
2200 O'Farrell
San Francisco, CA 94115
(415) 929-4000

University of California Hospitals and Clinics
513 Parnassus Avenue
San Francisco, CA 94143
(415) 666-9000

Stanford University Medical Center
300 Pasteur Drive
Stanford, CA 94305
(415) 497-2300

Harbor General Hospital
1000 W. Carson Street
Torrance, CA 90509
(213) 533-2104

Colorado

Fitzsimmons Army Medical Center
Peoria and Colfax streets
Denver, CO 80240
(303) 341-8281

National Asthma Center
1999 Julian Street
Denver, CO 80204
(303) 458-1999

National Jewish Hospital
3800 E. Colfax Avenue
Denver, CO 80206
(303) 388-4461

University of Colorado Medical Center
4200 E. Ninth Avenue
Denver, CO 80262
(303) 394-7601

Connecticut

Yale–New Haven Medical Center
333 Cedar Street
New Haven, CT 06510
(203) 436-8060

District of Columbia

Children's Hospital National Medical Center
111 Michigan Avenue
Washington, DC 20010
(202) 745-5000

Georgetown University Hospital
3800 Reservoir Road, N.W.
Washington, DC 20007
(202) 625-7001

Howard University Hospital
2041 Georgia Avenue, N.W.
Washington, DC 20060
(202) 745-1596

Florida

Division of Allergy and Immunology
University of South Florida
Tampa, FL 33612
(813) 972-2000

William A. Shands Teaching Hospital and Clinics
University of Florida
Gainesville, FL 32610
(904) 392-3771

Illinois

Institute of Allergy and Clinical Immunology
Grant Hospital of Chicago
550 W. Webster Avenue
Chicago, IL 60614
(312) 883-2000

Michael Reese Hospital and Medical Center
508 E. 29th Street
Chicago, IL 60616
(312) 791-2000

Northwestern University Memorial Hospital
Superior Street and Fairbanks Court
Chicago, IL 60611
(312) 649-8624

Rush-Presbyterian-St. Luke's Medical Center
1753 W. Congress Parkway
Chicago, IL 60612
(312) 942-5000

University of Illinois Hospital
1919 W. Taylor Street
Chicago, IL 60612
(312) 996-7000

Iowa

University of Iowa Hospitals and Clinics
650 Newton Road
Iowa City, IA 52242
(391) 356-1616

Kansas

University of Kansas College of Health Sciences and
Bell Memorial Hospital
39th Street and Rainbow Blvd.
Kansas City, KS 66103
(913) 588-6008

Louisiana

Tulane University School of Medicine
Allergy Clinic
1430 Tulane Avenue
New Orleans, LA 70112
(504) 588-5578

Maryland

Good Samaritan Hospital
5601 Lock Raven Blvd.
Baltimore, MD 21239
(301) 323-2200

Johns Hopkins Hospital
601 N. Broadway
Baltimore, MD 21205
(301) 955-5000

Massachusetts

Children's Hospital Medical Center
300 Longwood Avenue
Boston, MA 02115
(617) 734-6000

Massachusetts General Hospital
Clinical Immunology and Allergy Unit
Fruit Street
Boston, MA 02114
(617) 726-2000

Robert B. Brigham Hospital
125 Parker Hill Avenue
Boston, MA 02120
(617) 732-5055

Michigan

University Hospital
1405 E. Ann Street
Ann Arbor, MI 48109
(313) 764-3184

Henry Ford Hospital
2799 W. Grand Blvd.
Detroit, MI 48202
(313) 876-2600

Minnesota

University of Minnesota Hospitals and Clinics
516 Delaware Street
Minneapolis, MN 55455
(612) 373-8484

Mayo Clinic and Foundation
200 First Street, S.W.
Rochester, MN 55901
(507) 284-2511

Missouri

Children's Mercy Hospital
24th Street and Gillham Road
Kansas City, MO 64108
(816) 234-3000

Barnes Hospital—Washington University Medical School
Barnes Hospital Plaza
St. Louis, MO 63110
(314) 454-2000

St. Louis University Medical Center
1402 S. Grand Blvd.
St. Louis, MO 63104
(314) 664-9800

Nebraska

St. Joseph Hospital
601 N. 30th Street
Omaha, NB 68131
(402) 449-4001

New York

Jewish Hospital and Medical Center of Brooklyn
555 Prospect Place
Brooklyn, NY 11238
(212) 240-1761

Children's Hospital of Buffalo
219 Bryant Street
Buffalo, NY 14222
(716) 878-7000

Nassau County Medical Center
2201 Hempstead Tpk.
East Meadow, NY 11554
(516) 542-0123

R.A. Cooke Institute of Allergy—Roosevelt Hospital
428 W. 59th Street
New York, NY 10028
(212) 554-7000

Cornell Medical School—New York Hospital
510 E. 70th Street
New York, NY 10021
(212) 472-5900

New York University Medical Center
552 First Avenue
New York, NY 10016
(212) 340-5241

Strong Memorial Hospital of the University of Rochester
601 Elmwood Avenue
Rochester, NY 14642
(716) 275-2121

North Carolina

Duke University Medical Center
Durham, NC 27710
(919) 684-8111

Ohio

Children's Hospital Medical Center
Elland and Bethesda avenues
Cincinnati, OH 45229
(513) 559-4200

Cleveland Clinic Foundation
9500 Euclid Avenue
Cleveland, OH 44106
(216) 444-5780

Ohio State University Hospitals
456 Clinic Drive
Columbus, OH 43210
(614) 422-4851

Pennsylvania

Children's Hospital of Philadelphia
34th Street and Civic Center Blvd.
Philadelphia, PA 19104
(215) 596-9100

Hahnemann Medical College and Hospital
Feinstein Bldg.
216 N. Broad Street
Philadelphia, PA 19102
(215) 448-7000

Hospital of University of Pennsylvania
34th and Spruce streets
Philadelphia, PA 19104
(215) 662-4000

Thomas Jefferson University Hospital
11th and Walnut streets
Philadelphia, PA 19107
(215) 928-6000

Children's Hospital of Pittsburgh
125 De Soto Street
Pittsburgh, PA 15213
(412) 647-2345

Rhode Island

Rhode Island Hospital
593 Eddy Street
Providence, RI 02902
(401) 277-4000

Texas

University of Texas Medical Branch Hospitals
8th and Mechanic streets
Galveston, TX 77550
(713) 765-1011

Texas Children's Hospital—Baylor College of Medicine
6621 Fannin
Houston, TX 77030
(713) 791-4219

University of Texas Health Sciences Center
7703 Floyd Curl Drive
San Antonio, TX 78284
(512) 691-6011

Virginia

University of Virginia Hospitals
Private Clinic Bldg.
Hospital Drive
Charlottesville, VA 22908
(804) 924-0211

Medical College of Virginia Hospitals
12th and Marshall streets
Richmond, VA 23298
(804) 786-9000

Washington

University Hospital
1959 N.E. Pacific Street
Seattle, WA 98195
(206) 543-3300

Wisconsin

University of Wisconsin Hospital and Clinics
600 Highland Avenue
Madison, WI 53702
(608) 263-8000

Milwaukee County Medical Complex
8700 W. Wisconsin Avenue
Milwaukee, WI 53226
(414) 257-5915

APPENDIX J

Sources of Hypoallergenic Products for Allergic Children

Most specialized products for the allergic child can be found in your own local area. Depending on your child's particular needs, consult the classified telephone directory under the following headings:

Air Cleaning and Purifying Equipment
Air Pollution Control
Clean Rooms — Installation and Equipment
Dust and Fume Collecting Systems
Dust Control Materials
Environmental and Ecological Services
Health and Diet Food Products
Hospital Equipment and Supplies
Safety Equipment

In addition, most large, diversified mercantile chains (Sears, J.C. Penney, Montgomery Ward, etc.) stock some of the appliances or products allergic children require.

The following firms supply the products indicated under their names. The information should not be taken as an endorsement of any firm, product, or service listed. Additional suppliers of allergy products are listed in *Allergy Products Directory*, which has been compiled by the staff of the American Allergy Association. This valuable information source is available for $9.95 from

Allergy Publications Group
P.O. Box 640
Menlo Park, CA 94026

Your allergist or Health Maintenance Organization may also be able to point you to local sources of hypoallergenic products.

Air-Conditioning Engineers
211 Railroad
Blue Mound, IL
(217) 692-2812
Air cleaners and purifiers

All Around Allergy Products Company
P.O. Box 393
Bronxville, NY 10708
(914) 779-2400
Books; hypoallergenic toy animals; sleeping bags; bedding and bedding protectors; pillows; peak flow meters; inspiratory trainers; nebulizers; dust, mold, and mildew controls; various air cleaners, ionizers, humidifiers

Allergen-Proof Encasing
1450 E. 363rd Street
Eastlake, OH 44094
Bedding

Aller Guard
Medical Plaza Building
P.O. Box 58027
Topeka, KS 66658
(913) 233-0279
Mattress covers

Allergy Control Products
28 High Ridge Avenue
Ridgefield, CT 06877
Mattress and pillow encasings

The Allergy Store
7345 Healdsburg Avenue
Sebastopol, CA 95472
(800) 222-9090
(800) 824-7163 (outside California)
Bedding, air cleaners, humidifiers

The AL-R-G Shoppe, Inc.
3411 Johnson Street
Hollywood, FL 33021
(305) 981-9182
Books; bedding; dust, mold, and mildew controls; air cleaners; respiratory aids

Bio-Tech Systems
P.O. Box 25380
Chicago, IL 60625
(800) 621-5545
Air cleaners; mold spray; masks; bedding

Cloud 9 Air Purification Products
242 W. Devon Avenue
Bensenville, IL 60106
(312) 595-5700
Air cleaners

Collins Designers
Presidential House
317 Presidential Way
Guilderland, NY 12084
(518) 456-6845
Bedding

CRSI Environmental Systems
670 Mariner Drive
Michigan City, IN 46360
(800) 272-3786
Residential air purification systems

DeVilbiss Health Care Worldwide
P.O. Box 635
Somerset, PA 15501
(814) 443-4881
DeVilbiss Pulmo-Aide nebulizers

Dura Pharmaceuticals, Inc.
P.O. Box 28331
San Diego, CA 92128
(619) 789-6840
Dura Neb 2000 nebulizers

Energy Efficient Systems Assoc.
450 Smith Street
Middletown, CT 06457
(800) 622-3358
(800) 243-3482 (outside Connecticut)
Electronic air purifiers

Environmental Corporation
P.O. Box 31313
St. Louis, MO 63131
(314) 966-6686
Mattress covers

King-Aire
P.O. Box 149
Carmel, IN 46032
(317) 845-1170
(800) 368-3795 (outside Indiana)
Air cleaners

Mine Safety Appliance Co.
519 Niagara Street
Tonawanda, NY 14150
(716) 691-6922
Dustfoe 66 Respirator Mask

Newtron Products
1260 West Sharon Road
P.O. Box 18112
Cincinnati, OH 45218
(800) 543-9149
(513) 561-7373
Air cleaners

Index